T0146088

On Race and Medicine

On Race and Medicine

Insider Perspectives

Edited by Richard Garcia

ROWMAN & LITTLEFIELD
Lanham • Boulder • New York • London

Published by Rowman & Littlefield
A wholly owned subsidiary of The Rowman & Littlefield Publishing Group, Inc.
4501 Forbes Boulevard, Suite 200, Lanham, Maryland 20706
www.rowman.com

Unit A, Whitacre Mews, 26-34 Stannary Street, London SE11 4AB

British Library Cataloguing in Publication Information Available

Library of Congress Cataloging-in-Publication Data

On race and medicine : insider perspectives / edited by Richard Garcia.
p. ; cm.
Includes bibliographical references.
ISBN 978-1-4422-4835-9 (cloth : alk. paper) — ISBN 978-1-4422-4836-6 (electronic)
I. Garcia, Richard, 1964– , editor.
[DNLM: 1. Social Medicine—United States—Essays. 2. Health Status Disparities—United States—Essays. 3. Racism—United States—Essays. WA 31]
RA418
362.10973—dc23
2014048144

∞™ The paper used in this publication meets the minimum requirements of American National Standard for Information Sciences Permanence of Paper for Printed Library Materials, ANSI/NISO Z39.48-1992.

Printed in the United States of America

Contents

Part IV: Toward Solutions

Bebop—an Intro

Richard Garcia

Healthcare discussions are typically about cost, more or less. Excess cost for excess care is the intended distress signal. Certainly, no one is talking about cutting necessary medical care, but "trim the fat" is the tireless mantra that everyone—politician, health insurance executive, taxpayer, insured, uninsured, even the overweight—can peaceably chant together.

I thought of this book as an arc that would begin with the crushing evidence of health disparities based on race, and then bend toward solutions in the end. The first chapter would lead me into a nuanced, personal address of disparities in health based on race. Writers of the next chapters were to take on the clear, but daunting, assignment of narrating private, personal perspectives that could serve as public inspiration as we examined race in American medicine. My original take was that disparities—both health *status* and health *care*—based on race are subsets of generally poor healthcare quality (given the price we pay) in the United States. Countless journal articles, national medical reports, newspaper articles, speeches, panels, and private discussions on the topic run like a continuous-loop video.

I never thought the word "disparities" was adequate to frame how this topic could best be examined. The word clandestinely points to "parity," in the end, which isn't where I'm headed. But it's the word that seems to have stuck. All right, then: Black men with chest pain wait longer for an initial EKG than White men (the same is true for Hispanic men); both Black and Hispanic men with long bone fractures wait longer for a smaller dose of pain medication; Black infants die at a higher rate than White infants; lower limb amputations and blindness, as complications of diabetes, are highest among Hispanics; death among Black people is in excess; the Agency for Healthcare Research and Quality notes that Asian-Pacific Islanders are 16 percent more likely than Whites to die from serious but treatable complications in US hospitals; and so on.

1

I started writing this book with the following deduction, which seemed logical to me: America pays more for healthcare than any other country, and the quality of this healthcare (measured by various items like life expectancy, infant mortality, morbidity associated with common chronic diseases like diabetes, and the like) is far inferior when compared with other developed countries like Sweden, France, Germany, or Canada. If the United States spends more money than any other country, we ought to have better health results; if not, then we ought to decrease spending. Either way, sicker people cost more, and racial minorities are sicker, based upon *all* the evidence. So, people in the United States will save money if these disparities in health between the races are decreased, and even more money if they are eliminated. (Naturally, this argument is no good. If we had, say, the highest health outcomes quality on earth, we would not be satisfied, and the thrust would still be to decrease costs. Quality, it seems, isn't quite the issue.)

In the end, however, as I thought about this more, and collected the chapters in this book, I became convinced that I was wrong. Health disparities are *not* subsets of healthcare quality. That's why *that* book cannot be written.

Health *care* and health *status* appeared to me as the two overlapping circles of a Venn diagram. Related, interdependent, one partly embedded in the other. But the overlapping center—the sweet spot—does not enjoy the extraordinary attention that such diagrams set out to promote. That is to say, *all* areas are critical. Beyond this, the overlapping area is in flux. For example, always looming for a healthy patient are trauma, a new lump, or an imploding blood vessel in the brain. And for sick patients, there are treatment successes and failures that rearrange where their health status rests. They may need more or less care, with time. In other words, health, like time itself, is an all-at-once matter, in the present.

Health *status*—the medical condition in which we find ourselves, good or bad—and health *care*—the treatment we receive in the ER, from our own doctor, or from a healthcare "system," let's say—are related.

I recently underwent an "employment physical" where the doctor checked my throat and my ears, listened to an inspiration on the left side of my chest and an expiration on the right, briefly listened to my heart, and scarcely touched the skin on my abdomen. (He didn't even ask me to remove my shirt for this exam.) This is not wonderful healthcare. But I'm a physician, and healthy, I think. If the doctor missed any cancer because he didn't perform standard physical exams or order standard screening tests, then my health status will worsen. I could argue that this phantom cancer might have been identified early had the doctor bothered to check. (Given that cancer grows unchecked, I'll eventually find out either way, I'm afraid.)

Or consider a young man with a nagging wrist injury who, coincidentally, also had high blood pressure the day he visited his doctor. The doctor addressed the wrist injury, but not the high blood pressure. The doctor didn't mention the need for a subsequent blood pressure measurement to be sure that it was a transient elevation destined to return to normal. While the elevation wasn't extraordinary in this young Black man, sustained high blood pressure over many years is most preventable, but can be most expensive, and most deadly, if left untreated. Everyone in medicine understands this concept. But even though everyone understands this in medicine, the young Black man's elevated blood pressure was dismissed in favor of some other future, contiguous with an ignored past.

The healthcare in these two brief examples could render the middle-aged Mexican man and the young Black man sicker and in need of more expensive care in the years to come. Poor health *care* can lead to poor health *status*.

Or else the Mexican man will not get cancer, and the young Black man will get his blood pressure addressed soon enough by someone else. Either way, the healthcare cost will be higher than it could have been. I'm talking about the financial cost here. I'm not yet talking about the human cost. Who pays, and in what currency—cash or flesh—are items I'll examine later.

But *status* and *care* are also unrelated. Very sick patients usually receive wonderful care. And healthy patients usually receive good-enough preventive care, or none at all, which can suffice for the healthy person in the short run. This is the conundrum in which we find ourselves as we consider the quality of medicine available, and applied, in the United States. Naturally, when we add race to the mix, as in other areas of America, things become darker.

How is race related to healthcare? Before this question can be meaningfully placed, let alone answered, a more substantial question exists: *Why* is examining race in medicine even an issue worth the intellectual, if not the practical, effort?

Certainly, this book cannot be a whining collection that catalogs various inequalities, demonstrating connections to similar social and economic conditions in other components of American society, and asking for more and more that will do little to solve any problem at all. Then what can we say that establishes the exigency for people who are not obviously affected? What concrete betterment comes from these sorts of analyses? Better for whom? Who speaks for those with disparate health status, who receive lower *quality*—both product and service—of *care*?

Well, doctors do. All of us. This is our *raison d'être*, is it not?

It seems to me that a sincere attempt to decrease health disparities between races in America, like other complex topics that include race, requires a sincere consideration of the rhetorical triad: speaker, speech, audience.

The speakers' ethos—study, training, research, credentials, and esprit—licenses us to stand up and address race in medicine. Then there's the speech itself. What will we offer in place of yet another catalog of previously published racial differences in health status and healthcare, or a handful of would-be solutions that cannot decrease the disparities?

When we began to develop this book, some of the authors met in a house in Northern California and sat together to discuss our prospective chapters. While I knew everyone, the other authors didn't know each other as of yet. We told our fellow contributors what we intended to write, listened to everyone's intentions, and offered suggestions all around. Near the end of the first morning, Rick Rigsby caught me on the periphery of the group and said, "This book is going to be a mess. But a wonderful mess."

The reason this book promises to be such a "mess" is because we are writing *forensic* chapters that challenge the *way* disparities have been evaluated during the past decade or two.

Disparities in medicine based on race are medical staples requiring physicians, per se, to address them in substantive, life-saving ways. This is the route I took when I initially entered the "field" of health disparities. I then considered other arenas of race in American matters. That is, we could be law school professors and talk about disparities on death row or the adjudication rates between races; or professors in the school of education and talk about the disparities in public schools for minority children; or business school professors and talk about redlining and glass ceilings; and so forth. I imagine the topic of health disparities as a section in a syllabus of an American studies course, along with the other sections that consider race in America.

Race in medicine recapitulates race in America.

Then, physicians require the help of our colleagues in other fields of study: literature, anthropology, sociology, communications, business, and the rest. This is who we have here. While they are all my friends, this team of authors isn't haphazard. Nor is it interdisciplinary as a matter of convenience. The afflictions in medicine are integrated with our country's history, and its present, such that serious attention *requires* the vascular surgeon and the poet, the cardiologist and the rhetorician, the insurance executive and the sociologist, the pediatrician and the writer.

I thought I might become a pediatrician when I entered college mainly because someone asked me about my plans. I'd never considered any career at all until that moment when I answered the question asked by someone I cannot now remember. Much later, and with much less consideration, I thought I might also become a writer. I live a risky present as an educated adult, though now that my wife and children depend on a more thoughtful approach to life, I try to be better than I might have predicted from those primordial thoughts about what I might ever be.

My father's brother—my uncle, then—whom I've never met, is the champion jazz trumpet player in the entire state of California penitentiary system, from what I hear. I have no way of verifying this claim. Nor do I question it. I do, however, recognize my place on earth: a man from a long line of criminal men, on the one hand, and a doctor interested in race in America, on the other. I suppose I could simply work as a pediatrician, which was my dream. (Before he died from complications of obesity and ethos, my dearest friend, a rhetorician, pointed out to me how rare it is for anyone—especially someone from my childhood depths—to realize his dream.)

In my case, I thought my way out of my family and my neighborhood into a career in medicine precisely to prove to children like me that they are wrong about having to remain there. When I came back, I found that I was less interested in the clinical aspects of medicine, and more interested in an examination of race insofar as it clashes with medicine. Before I understood where I was in the matter, I'd written some articles, given some speeches, and passively, I must admit, found myself here, working in concert with some great thinkers on the topic.

I'm mindful that more and better descriptions of health disparities based on race promise to be tiresome for the audience. Alas, I'm certain that *solutions* to these disparities are in demand by the reader. But before anyone can produce such a prescription, a *forensic* book, I submit, is in order. That is, a jazz collective of thinkers, doctors, and writers apprising the discourse heretofore, and offering a response to the call, could be of some use. So, the next book on the Civil War, for example, will not end with a win for the South. *On Race and Medicine: Insider Perspectives* will not improve my mother's diabetes or get my brother, who has not seen a physician other than me since 1984, to see another one. This book won't get the next Mexican with chest pain a better consultation. And for Black people, it won't decrease the excess deaths that are easily and repeatedly documented in medical article after medical article.

My pediatrician from the 1960s was the only doctor on the entire side of my childhood city. He retired after forty-eight years in an office on the corner across the street from my high school. I was to follow him in his mission to work there, where he was most needed. But instead I'm here, where I hope to imbue his work with my own. He and I are different, it's true. We do agree that the constancy of disparities that he's seen throughout his career, and that I've noted in my own, leaves us in that place where race in America, and race in medicine, leads us: worse off than we can tolerate. But the speech of equality or fairness in medicine is anemic without a full-bodied, complicated audience. An audience interested in some personal essays that ask them, at least, to be willing to take a second—if not a first—closer look at race and medicine. What's more important than who we are, or what we say in these chapters, is how all this will be heard by the third, and most important, branch of the rhetorical triad: the audience.

These chapters hope to illuminate what neither social science nor medicine alone can tell us about the health of various racial and ethnic groups in America. These scholars from various disciplines—who don't ordinarily collaborate—write from their own disciplinary stances and particular points of view, and, in the end, they form a collective that, at once, considers the personal and the collective.

Here exists a different focus and intent than can be easily found in traditional medical and social scientific literatures. Some contributors focus on questions of "race"—what it is, and what it is not—while others consider the relationship between their own experiences and the broader issue of race and health disparities. Still others consider the personal essay itself as an instrument in a dialogue about race and medicine that is timely in American discourse.

The vascular surgeon offers his ordinarily inner thoughts about how he might help a doomed patient. A rhetorician considers how patients and physicians talk as he remembers his childhood pediatrician's house calls in Vallejo, California, while his wife dies in the present. An English professor considers his Mexicanness, then and now. A White cardiologist recognizes that his perception is based in unreality, and is surprised to find that well-meaning physicians, in fact, treat patients differently based on race. He then wonders how unsuspecting, well-meaning physicians can perpetuate disparities even when they believe they're treating everyone with the same, highest medical standards.

Scholars and physicians in this volume come from many fields, each one writing in the personal essay form, which allows a kind of thinking that provides unique contributions to traditional medical writings about health disparities based on race. These authors understand that no book—not this one, and not any before or after it—will close the gap in health disparities based on race in the United States any more than the next book on the Middle East will result in peace. Bringing these essays together, however, provides the rare opportunity for an honestly interdisciplinary perspective on questions surrounding race and health disparities.

While sociologists and anthropologists have long argued that race is a social and historical construction, race remains a biological unreality embedded in thinking, and actual care, in medicine. Here, we have all attempted what Richard Rodriguez calls "the autobiography of an idea," as told using the first-person singular pronoun: I.

Part I

Health Disparities

What is the social context of health disparities? How should this be included in discussions about disparities, their origins, and their end? Brian Smedley, lead author of the 2002 Institute of Medicine report *Unequal Treatment*, notes that more than a decade later nothing has materially changed. Smedley considers the social realities of his childhood city, Detroit, as he navigates the commensurate healthcare realities that are necessarily derived from neighborhoods lacking even basic social accoutrements. Troy Duster also offers a social scientific analysis of whether health disparities are a matter of genes or environment.

ONE

No Accident

Brian D. Smedley

When I was growing up in Detroit in the 1960s, grocery stores were abundant. I couldn't walk more than a few blocks in any direction from our home on Northlawn, near the intersection of Six Mile and Livernois Roads, without coming across an A&P Supermarket, a Farmer Jack, or a Kroger grocery store. We would go to any of these stores specifically because of the variety and quality of foods: A&P had the best produce, Farmer Jack the best beef, and so on.

That was a different Detroit than it is today. In the mid-1960s, African Americans, many of whom held steady jobs with the major automobile manufacturers, began integrating neighborhoods such as our west-side community. We moved to the Bagley neighborhood, just west of Palmer Park, around 1965, along with many other Black families who sought to own the neatly maintained two-family homes that dotted the landscape.

By 1966 and 1967, even a small child like me couldn't help but notice some dramatic changes: Homes were rapidly going up for sale, sometimes every third or fourth house. Moving vans loaded and unloaded every day, on every block. Our White friends were leaving. By 1970 there was one White child left in my second-grade class at Bagley Elementary School.

My family moved from Detroit in 1971, not to escape the neighborhood but to relocate to Boston for a new job opportunity for my mother. We returned every year to see family, but the old neighborhood was

11

dramatically different. By the mid-1970s, Whites were hard to find in formerly integrated west-side Detroit. Real estate agents no longer bothered to show homes in the city to White families, instead taking them (by request or by default) to Farmington Hills, Southfield, and other suburban communities that had yet to see a large influx of African Americans. White flight to the inner-ring Detroit suburbs didn't last long; today, Southfield and many other close-in suburbs are overwhelmingly Black.

I wouldn't suggest that all of the White families who left did so because of racial animus; some undoubtedly did, while others left for reasons that were racially "neutral," but nonetheless had racial undertones. Some saw that home values were slipping as a result of the quick pace of home turnover. Others might have been concerned about the quality of Detroit's public schools. Still others might have been unnerved by Detroit's 1967 and 1968 riots, which were sparked by persistent racism across many sectors, and by Dr. Martin Luther King's assassination.

The result was a self-perpetuating cycle of racial and class isolation that, while not unique to Detroit, hit the city and metro area very hard. Whites, who already had higher levels of education, income, and wealth, could escape to suburbs where they enjoyed better opportunities than the African Americans left behind in Detroit—better schools, nicer homes, better access to capital, and the like. These advantages allowed them to advance further up the socioeconomic ladder, while African Americans in Detroit found that their homes appreciated in value at a much slower pace (if they appreciated at all), that their neighbors were poorer, and that businesses began to close. Between 2000 and 2010, a quarter-million people left the city. Even grocery stores were harder to find.

This, I believe, was no accident.

Grocers, like anyone else in business, want to make a profit. They make the most profit in communities with the most money. Increasingly, this was not Detroit. It got to the point where there were no major grocery stores or supermarkets in Detroit for many years in the 1990s and early 2000s. Only a few are operating in the city today. Again, this is not a decision made overtly out of racial animus. But because segregation is so stark in the city, these kinds of daily decisions have racial consequences.

Today, in a typical Black neighborhood in Detroit, the most readily accessible and affordable foods are highly processed, high-fat, and high-sugar and/or high-sodium products, sold in carryout stores and fast-food restaurants or convenience stores. Finding fresh fruits and vegetables requires more effort. Preparing them requires even more effort.

And yet we wonder why so many people of color suffer from a host of chronic illnesses that could be prevented through proper nutrition. From the cradle to the grave, African Americans such as those living in Detroit suffer disproportionately from obesity-related illnesses such as diabetes, heart disease, some forms of cancer, arthritis—the list is long.

To compound the problem, we ask our healthcare systems to "fix" the health inequalities resulting from inequitable social, economic, and environmental conditions, such as limited access to healthy foods. Read any newspaper story on health disparities, or listen to most elected officials' comments on the issue, and one is left with the clear impression that it is the lack of access to high-quality healthcare that *causes* health inequalities.

Even if it were the case that US healthcare could reverse disease, how can our healthcare systems—which are replete with examples of inefficiency, inconsistent quality, and skyrocketing costs—address deep and persistent racial health inequalities? This is the question at the core of this book. There are no easy answers or simple policy prescriptions. Only complexity. This book explores this complexity, and offers surprising insights.

Many years after leaving Detroit, I had the privilege of working at the Institute of Medicine (IOM) as director of a study on healthcare disparities requested by Congress. The project presented a challenging question: Do people of color receive a lower quality of healthcare than Whites, even when access-related factors, such as health insurance or income, are equal?

In many respects, the question is an artificial one. There are few instances when circumstances are "equal" in all respects for White and minority patients. Anyone who's ventured into an inner-city hospital quickly realizes that these institutions are dealing with the collateral consequences of segregation and inequality, even among minority patients who are relatively well-off.

But the question is important because it focuses our attention on the relevance of race in what many people would assume is the most egalitarian space in America—the hospital or doctor's office. Healthcare professionals do the work they do because they care deeply about people. They seek to eliminate human suffering. And they presumably do so regardless of the patient's race, ethnicity, nationality, age, sexual orientation, gender, ability status, or other personal characteristics.

The IOM committee began its work by carefully reviewing the large body of research on healthcare disparities. (We began this review in 2000, resulting in the 2002 publication *Unequal Treatment*; today this literature is vastly expanded.) Many of the studies that we identified didn't meet the committee's criteria requiring careful control of, or adjustment for, racial differences in patient income, education, or insurance status. But of those that did, a clear pattern emerged: Regardless of the disease area, type of clinical procedure, or healthcare delivery setting, racial and ethnic minority patients received a lower quality of care than Whites. This was the finding of the overwhelming majority of studies. Critics argued that "publication bias" favored studies finding disparities. But in this area of research, bias could also—and perhaps as easily—work the other way, because published studies finding no disparities were rare, and could provide clues for intervention strategies.

Without question, patients are treated differently based on race and ethnicity. But is at least some of this difference clinically justified? The IOM *Unequal Treatment* report concluded that racial and ethnic differences in treatment response are modest at best, particularly given that racial and ethnic groups are much more genetically and biologically diverse within the groups than between them. Minority patients have been found to be more reluctant than White patients to accept physicians' recommendations—but in the most rigorous studies, the influence of patient preferences is modest. And clinical uncertainty on the part of healthcare providers—who may lack the cultural and linguistic proficiency to fully understand patients' presenting problems—also plays a role.

The kinds of differences in healthcare treatment and outcomes *not* due to these factors, *Unequal Treatment* stated, are disparities that are *unacceptable*. The IOM concluded that at least some of these disparities are the result of providers' biases and stereotypes, the overwhelming majority of which are unconscious or implicit: They are activated quickly and without awareness, and most often in conditions of time pressure and resource constraints. Implicit biases subtly encourage providers to fall back upon well-rehearsed cognitive scripts. And they do so in ways that shape behavior—a growing body of studies demonstrates that implicit bias among healthcare providers changes the way they respond to hypothetical case vignettes of patients from different racial and ethnic groups who are identical in all other respects.

Perhaps the most important source of healthcare disparities, in my view, is the persistent phenomenon of separate and unequal healthcare. While we've made great strides in desegregating hospitals, the reality in America is that there is a profound misalignment of healthcare resources relative to community need. Our poorest and minority communities are often our sickest communities, yet they face significant geographic barriers to healthcare. Few providers can afford to practice in these communities, and while the federal Health Resources and Services Administration has admirably sought to correct this imbalance through community health centers, health professions programs, and many other efforts to support the healthcare safety net, too many low-income and minority communities face a dearth of providers and hospitals.

To compound these problems, providers and institutions serving low-income communities are more likely than those in more advantaged communities to lack the resources and connections with specialists and academic health centers that might help their patients receive the highest quality of healthcare.

These structural inequities in healthcare delivery closely correspond to residential segregation. The average African American lives in a community where about 60 percent of his neighbors are also minorities. Over half of Hispanics live with minority neighbors. In contrast, over eight of every ten neighbors of Whites are White, on average.

My point is that the financing and delivery of healthcare is very much like other aspects of American life: Race and place powerfully shape access to health resources and risks, whether they are healthcare, food, environmental exposures, or neighborhood poverty.

And I don't mean to pick on Detroit—its city and county health agencies are working hard to reverse these health inequities, and community-based initiatives, such as Wayne County's Place Matters initiative, are helping to empower communities to address the conditions that shape health. Many other US cities suffer from the same problems of white flight, segregation, and poverty concentration. The result is that the health of people who live in neighborhoods left behind suffers. It's important that we draw attention to these root causes and point to strategies that work to improve opportunities for good health among people who've systematically faced barriers to good health. Our message should be a clear one: *Place* matters for health as a result of many complex and interacting factors, including access to healthcare.

The Detroit metro area is still one of the most segregated locales in the United States. Using a measure called the "dissimilarity index," demographers have calculated that 86 percent of African American and White residents of the Detroit metro area would have to move to create a completely integrated community. At the same time, the city has suffered from a dramatic population loss—fewer people, Black or White, choose to live in the city, while many more have no choice but to stay.

Detroit's problems won't be solved by the next election cycle. It may take ten years, fifteen years, or a generation to undo the inequities that have evolved over many past generations. While the nation has made great strides toward the elimination of racial inequality, this work is unfinished. Until it is completed, many people of color will suffer from poorer health and shortened life spans relative to White Americans. Importantly, we have the power to change these trends—they are not immutable. Doing so will not only improve the health of minority Americans but also make the nation as a whole fairer and more equitable for all.

TWO

Explaining Health Disparities

Is It Genes or Environment?

Troy Duster

I have never been comfortable with "health disparities" as a framework for addressing different rates of illness and health. An obvious reason is on the surface, but there is a subtler analytic reason that this frame partially obscures.

The obvious reason: In early 2006, the *New York Times* ran a four-part series on the soaring rates of Type II diabetes. One of the articles reported that rates of diabetes above 95th Street on the east side of Manhattan are at least three times the rates south of the dividing line.[1] The health disparities so noted could be reduced by increasing diabetes below 95th Street. But the reduced gap would please no one. If health disparities reduction based upon an accelerating rate of diabetes among the middle classes seems forced or counterintuitive, consider the fact that in India, the diabetes rate among the middle classes has soared in the last two decades—placing the well-to-do at far greater risk for this disease than the poorest part of the population. No one wants to see the gap closed by a parallel soaring rate of diabetes among India's poor. To put it bluntly, then, reducing health disparities is not the goal, but reducing diabetes most certainly is!

But there is a second, more subtle reason for jettisoning health disparities as the conceptual framework for an approach to health issues, and

17

Richard Garcia alludes to this in his introductory essay. Why would we expect health and illness outcomes sorted by race in medicine to be anything else but a reflection of race in the larger society? The analogy to our extremely racialized prison population makes the point quite sharply. As with health disparities, rates of incarceration are notably different by race. Why would we expect outcomes by race in criminal justice to be anything else but a reflection of race in the larger society? To reduce "incarceration rate disparities," we could embark on a program to increase the number and proportion of Whites and Asians who are imprisoned—but while that has heuristic and rhetorical uses, it is not a strategy anyone can seriously advocate. So, again, the issue is not to reduce prison-rate disparities, but to reduce crime! Exhorting potential consumers to "just say no" to drugs has had little effect upon the four-fold increase in our prison population of the last three decades.[2] Similarly, in a society in which race has long been a stratifying practice that structurally reinforces the political and economic domination of one group, increasing the health of the poor will involve so much more than exhortations to eat healthier and get more exercise.

The question of how best to approach a strategy to increase the health of the disenfranchised and economically distressed is a hotly contested issue, mainly because of the overlap of poverty, illness, ethnicity, and race. This overlap has led some to conclude that there is something basically different in the biogenetic makeup of different groups that might explain health disparities. The Pima Indians have a very high rate of diabetes, and they have become the subject of intense scrutiny and research as to why. Here is an excerpt from an account of the approach supported by the National Institutes of Health that I have termed elsewhere "looking inside the body"[3] for answers:

> Beginning in 1983 and continuing for 10 years, the National Institute of Diabetes and Digestive and Kidney Diseases (NIDDK) studied the genetic codes of almost 300 non-diabetic Pima Indians in great detail. "We looked at body composition, how well a person produced insulin, how well that person's cells responded to insulin, and other factors. After a number of years, some of the volunteers developed diabetes and we were able to determine that insulin resistance and obesity were major predictors of disease," Dr. Bogardus explains.
>
> Because diabetes is such a complex disease, Dr. Bogardus and his staff are attempting to narrow their search by first looking for the genetic causes of physical conditions that can lead to diabetes, such as the

genes that influence a person's cells to secrete less and respond less to insulin that is needed to regulate blood sugar.

In 1993, they identified a gene called FABP2 that may contribute to insulin resistance. This gene makes an intestinal fatty acid binding protein using one of two amino acids. When the gene makes the protein with threonine, one of those amino acids, the body seems to absorb more fatty acids from the fat in meals. NIH scientists think that could lead to a higher level of certain fats and fatty acids in the blood, which could contribute to insulin resistance. [4]

Of known potentially effective interventions, this approach does not have (indeed, could not have) much of a track record. For at least the last half century, we have known that the rate of Type II diabetes among Native Americans is more than double that of Whites in the United States.

Until quite recently, the dominant theory among geneticists who have approached this topic has strongly suggested that Native Americans are far more likely to possess genes that enable fat-hoarding, sometimes labeled "thrifty genes." They hypothesized that these genes were conducive to adaptation because their ancestors had a need to survive during cycles of famine. However, since this group now lives in a world in which they can routinely ingest foods with high fat and sugar content, these putatively formerly protective/adaptive genes are now placing this population at greater risk for diabetes.

A recent study suggests that it was the high-fiber diet that "locked into place" the thrifty genes, not the adaptive mechanisms generated by famine cycles. [5] Notice that in both accounts, genes play a dominant role in explaining "health disparities." Yet we have strong evidence that diet has far more analytic explanatory power, across all groups, when addressing the diabetes crisis that has spread across the globe since 1980. The fastest rate of increase is in India, which the World Health Organization has called the diabetes capital of the world. Current estimates suggest that at least thirty-five million in India suffer from the disease now, and best estimates predict this figure will double in the next decade. [6] As noted earlier, the growing middle classes of India are far more likely to get the disease, and "thrifty genes" have less to do with this than the recent capacity of the newly wealthy to consume high levels of sugar in the countless ceremonies and ritual dinner celebrations the new middle classes can now afford.

Table 2.1. Prevalence of Diabetes in *Related* Populations

	Traditional	Prevalence (%)	Westernized	Prevalence (%)
Amerindians	Mapuche	0	Pima	23
New Guinea	Rural	0	Urban	37
Australian Aborigines	Rural	0	Urban	23
Middle East	Yemen	4	Lebanon	14
Chinese	Rural China	0	Urban Taiwan	13
Asian Indian	Rural India	0	Fiji	22

H. King and M. Rewers, "Global Estimates for Prevalence of Diabetes Mellitus and Impaired Glucose Tolerance," *Diabetes Care* 16 (1993): 157–77.

To return to the extraordinarily high rate of diabetes among the Pima, a very different approach sets the analytic frame in a broader socio-historical context. Those who approach the matter from this angle have a very different view of how to think about diabetes prevention and treatment. In table 2.1, note the striking pattern of urban versus rural dwelling among six populations across the globe.[7] The Pima who live in urban areas have an exceedingly high rate of diabetes, but those who live in "traditional" sites where they practice "traditional culture" hardly experience any diabetes.

Of course, what is striking about this table is that this pattern holds true for every group sampled, across a wide swath of the globe. Did they all have thrifty genes, and, if so, what intervention is implied other than a dramatic shift in diet? Or, from another perspective, since the sharp increase in Type II diabetes has come about in the last three decades, just in pure scientific logic, far more of the variance is explained by a systematic empirical investigation of shifting patterns of nutritional intake. Can one even seriously hypothesize that the Indian middle classes' higher incidence is best explained by their genes versus the combination of increased wealth and attendant cultural norms that require a plethora of sugar-laden pastries at every ritual, holiday, birthday, wedding, and so forth?

CANCER AND HEALTH DISPARITIES BETWEEN RACIALLY AND ETHNICALLY DESIGNATED POPULATIONS

One-half of all cancers occur among people living in the industrialized world, although this group constitutes only one-fifth of the world's population.[8] The World Health Organization collected data on cancer rates from seventy countries and came to the conclusion that at least 80 percent of all cancer is attributable to environmental influences.[9] It is possible that both reporting problems and earlier deaths in the rest of the world may explain some of these differences, but migrant studies are among the most powerfully persuasive devices that can be used to sharpen and isolate the environmental sources behind the high incidence of cancer.

Migrants to Australia, Canada, Israel, and the United States all illustrate this pattern. Consider Jewish women who migrate from North Africa, where breast cancer is rare, to Israel, a nation with a high incidence. Initially, their breast cancer risk is one-half that of their Israeli counterparts. But within thirty years, African-born and Israeli-born Jews show identical breast cancer rates.[10]

In one of the most compelling environmental studies of cancer ever conducted, researchers found a statistically significant association between the use of agricultural chemicals and cancer mortality in 1,497 rural US counties.[11]

In the United States, the rate of prostate cancer for African Americans is double that for White Americans. If we begin with these figures—and have no sense of history, sociology, or epidemiology—then it would seem legitimate to ask the scientific question: Is "race" as a biological concept playing a role? Indeed, just as there are molecular geneticists searching for genes that predispose Aborigines and Native Americans to alcohol abuse by looking only inside the body, there are those looking for an answer to higher rates of prostate cancer among Blacks—the search for what are called "candidate genes" in this "special population."

But a far more plausible explanation comes from an analysis of the sustained structural location of US Blacks, derived from more than three and a half centuries with a predominant social location at the base of the US economic structure. A sharply higher proportion of Blacks live in poverty, and they are many more times as likely to reside near toxic waste sites.[12]

THE GLOBAL REACH OF EXPLAINING HEALTH DISPARITIES
RESEARCH BY RACE AND ETHNICITY[13]

In 2009, the HUGO Pan-Asian SNP Consortium, an international research team led by Edison Liu of the Genome Institute of Singapore, mapped genetic variation and migration patterns in seventy-three Asian populations, with data coming from ten Asian countries: Japan, Korea, China, Taiwan, Singapore, Indonesia, the Philippines, Malaysia, Thailand, and India.[14] The results—which included a summary statement that "there is substantial genetic proximity of SEA (Southeast Asian) and EA (East Asian) populations"—were published in the journal *Science*.[15] In the same year, the Iressa Pan-Asian study (IPASS) was carried out by researchers in Hong Kong, China, Taiwan, Thailand, and Japan with the participation of eighty-seven centers in nine countries in Asia.[16]

The explicit, heightened racial consciousness of data reporting in human genomic science was dramatically on display in the November 6, 2008, issue of *Nature*. That journal published two articles, asserting triumphantly how, for the first time, the whole human genomes of "an Asian individual" and of a Yoruban—"an African individual"—were now "revealed." Here is an excerpt from the first article:

> Here we present the first diploid genome sequence of an Asian individual. . . . We aligned the short reads onto the NCBI human reference genome to 99.97% coverage, and guided by the reference genome, we used uniquely mapped reads to assemble a high-quality consensus sequence for 92% of the Asian individual's genome.[17]

Then, remarkably, *Nature* issued a press briefing stating:

> The . . . paper reports the genome of an Asian individual . . . Jian Wang and colleagues illustrate the potential of personal genomics in disease diagnosis, and by comparing this genome with the other individual genomes already available, those of J.D. Watson and J.C. Venter, they are able to shed light on the genetic variation in individuals of different ethnicity.

The press report refers to the fact that both James D. Watson, Nobel Prize winner as codiscoverer of the DNA molecule, and Craig Venter, head of the private sector group that codeveloped the map of the human genome, have had their full genomes sequenced. Both are White males. But why employ this particular taxonomic system to try to sort out useful, important, or relevant "differences"? The answer lies in a closer examination of recent emerging scientific discourse about "ancestral populations" and the fluid and contested boundaries around what constitutes a "population."

At the end of the twentieth century, the first draft of the Human Genome Map was completed, providing two kinds of hope for the near future. The first was quite explicitly about potential medical advances—that the completed map would spur the development of new kinds of therapies that would increase health and reduce the ravages of a wide variety of diseases. The second hope was more of a diffuse political aspiration, but it was loudly trumpeted at the famous White House news conference in June 2000. President Bill Clinton (US), Prime Minister Tony Blair (UK), and the two molecular geneticists who had led the public and private sector human genome projects all agreed on one thing: *At the level of DNA, there is no such thing as race.*

However, this pronouncement about the "end" of race echoes Mark Twain, who once quipped, in response to a newspaper's report that he had died, "The news of my death has been greatly exaggerated." So it has been with racial and ethnic categories. Indeed, there is substantial evidence that developments in several fields of inquiry relevant to molecular genetics (pharmacogenomics, pharmacotoxicology, clinical genetics, and forensic science) have actually served to reinscribe race as a biological category.[18]

Inadvertently, governments in industrializing nations are now aiding this development. Indeed, one of the most striking developments of the last few years has been the move by several governments to take strong protective "ownership" of the DNA of their own populations—a move designed to protect from possible bio-piracy carried out by the pharmaceutical industry in Western countries. Ruha Benjamin has called this "national genomic sovereignty," and it represents the opposite of the universal notion of human DNA envisaged at the completion of the Human Genome Project.[19]

On the surface, this policy frame asserts a deeply nationalist sentiment of self-determination in a time of increasing globalization. It implicitly "brands" national populations as biologically distinct from other populations, "naturalizing" nation-state boundaries to ensure that less powerful countries receive the economic and medical benefits that may result from population genomics.[20]

Mexico amended its General Health Law in 2008 to make "the sampling of genetic material and its transport outside of Mexico without prior approval . . . illegal."[21] The Genomic Sovereignty amendment states that Mexican-derived human genome data are the property of Mexico's government, and prohibits and penalizes its collection and utilization in research without prior government approval. It seeks to prevent other nations from analyzing Mexican genetic material, especially when results can be patented, and comes with a formidable bite in the form of prison time and lost wages.[22]

Mexico may be in the vanguard in being so explicit in asserting its commitment to national "genomic sovereignty," but the nation is hardly alone. India, China, Thailand, and South Africa have all issued policy statements or passed legislation designed to develop national genomics infrastructures to benefit their populations.[23] Thus we see a shifting emphasis in the last decade, sharply distinct from the original framing of the Human Genome Project. Rather than promoting the view that "we are all basically the same" at the DNA level, governments in these industrializing nations have begun to emphasize their populations' genetic uniqueness and are constructing strong protective political boundaries around access to that uniqueness. In so doing, while trying to fend off the potential for bio-piracy that they see as characterizing Western pharmaceutical companies' recent history, they are simultaneously slipping into the discourse of national (ethnic) and racial genetic categories. To show how these categories are coproduced by scientific and political concerns, it will be instructive to turn briefly to a history of the evolving taxonomies.

From the mid-nineteenth century to the present, both the categories of race and the social processes that reinforce the stratification of those racial categories (racism) have undergone significant changes. At various points in the last 150 years, scientists have used taxonomic systems that included as many as thirty different races, and they have pursued research programs designed to show the biological basis of those differences. In terms of social and political processes, racist behavior has been dramatically transformed from the early and crude behavior of lynch mobs to the legally institutionalized development of separate public facilities. The most egregious form, racial apartheid in South Africa, ended nearly two decades ago. While these crude forms have dissipated, as we shall see, race and racism have "morphing capacities"—the ability to take different shapes and substance.

For example, the last decade—the era of human molecular genetics and DNA analyses—has witnessed the emergence of new debates about the appropriate use of race in clinical medicine and scientific research in terms of the appropriate administration of pharmaceuticals to different "ancestral populations." A number of population geneticists, molecular biologists, and clinical practitioners are advocating that race should be deployed as a crude proxy for ancestry in prescribing drugs.[24]

IRESSA—LUNG CANCER AND ASIANS

The British firm AstraZeneca conducted a large clinical trial across the full population of patients suffering from advanced stages of lung cancer to test the efficacy of one of its most promising drugs, Iressa. The drug was first introduced in 2002, and over 45,000 patients worldwide have since taken Iressa. It is designed to treat the most common form of lung cancer by blocking an enzyme that otherwise causes cancer cells to proliferate. In the full study, the difference between those on a placebo and those taking Iressa was statistically insignificant. When the results were announced, the FDA began reviewing the situation to determine whether the drug should be pulled from the market. However, in re-reviewing the data by race and ethnicity, it was determined that while 5.5 was the average number of months of life prolonged for the general population, Asians had a 9.5-month prolongation, nearly double the average. Immediately, AstraZeneca touted the findings as significant, and the company began ramping up for shifting its marketing strategies and sales to Asian countries.[25]

Two elements now combine in a synergistic way to set the stage for the "hurricane just offshore," waiting for the winds to change. The first centers on new diagnostic technologies of bio-informatics, computer-assisted analysis of patterns of DNA. The second concerns new research on specific populations and allele frequency markers for those populations that just happen to occasionally coincide with socially defined groupings that we used to call ethnic and racial groupings, but are now increasingly referred to as those aggregated by "population-specific allelic frequency patterns." With new computers, we can now put the DNA of several clusters of people on computer chips and see what might be patterns in their DNA.[26]

We can do that with hundreds, even thousands of experiments in a few hours. Sometimes this proves to be a useful technology in the hunt for particular regions that might help explain some illnesses. One strategy for clinical genetics—to find "candidate genes" for a particular condition for those who suffer from a similar illness (for example, prostate cancer)—would be to obtain the tissue samples of several hundred patients with prostate cancer, and then look for patterns in their SNP profiles using this chip technology. With these new SNP profiles, it is possible that a researcher, driven not by a theoretical question but simply by sorting through those profiles entered into the forensic database, will come up with new taxonomies of people who share certain kinds of patterns in their DNA.

But what happens when rates of prostate cancer differ significantly among groups that have been racially designated? This way of framing the problem leaves one vulnerable to making a profoundly subtle interpretive error: By holding other factors constant (statistically, such as income, education, class, etc.) and finding persisting racial differences, one has substantial grounds for concluding that race is more biological than it is social and political.

HOW TO DEFINE A "POPULATION" FOR THE PURPOSES OF GENETIC RESEARCH

"Populations" are, as Fujimura and Rajagopalan noted, "both the production and outcomes of these [genome-wide association] studies."[27] Moreover, as Benjamin has demonstrated, "societies employ numerous types of classificatory schemes to sort and hierarchize populations, so that analyses about the ways in which race, nation, genomics, and identity are co-constituted in the Euro-American context are not readily transplantable to societies with very different histories of social-group-making."[28] Populations designated by genetic markers are most likely to become the subject of pharmaceutical inquiry and focus.

Drug firms, private biotech firms, and university medical centers are surely now poised to build DNA chips and engage in the business of genetic testing for drug effectiveness, based upon emerging definitional boundaries of "populations." Friedrich notes that "the Commission approved the marketing of gefitinib (Iressa) for selected patients with non-small cell lung cancer . . . the key ingredient in the commission's approval is patient selection—the proviso that gefitinib be used only in patients with certain mutations in the epidermal growth factor receptor (EGFR) gene that make them sensitive to the drug."[29] Tony Mok, the principal investigator of IPASS, advocates EGFR mutation testing when talking about the clinical implications of the IPASS study:

> In the past, all patients diagnosed with lung cancer would take chemotherapy, but not all of them would benefit. Now our study has shown that gefitinib is more efficacious on lung cancer patients with EGFR mutation. The new paradigm is that doctors may check for EGFR mutation and prescribe a personalized treatment plan for the appropriate patient.[30]

In sharp contrast, Cheng suggests that "the use of gene mutations as a predictable factor for practice is not feasible."[31] Kolata reports that "these so-called targeted therapies are only as good as tests to find their protein targets. And while most patients do not yet know it, those tests can be surprisingly unreliable. . . . [For example] those tests, for estrogen receptors on breast cancer cells, determine whether cancer will be thwarted by drugs that deprive tumors of estrogen. They can be wrong at least 10 percent of the time."[32]

Hovering over all of these developments is, certainly, the fluid determination of the relevant "population" in which to locate the right patient.

Tangwisutijit suggests that Thailand's involvement in the Pan-Asian SNP Consortium could mean that "ethnic groups living in isolated communities would not understand what the researchers told them when taking blood samples, and that the urban populations might be vulnerable to pharmacogenomic research, as they might unwittingly become guinea pigs for new medications."[33] Most recently, the Havasupai ruling in the United States—where a university settled a claim with a population on the misuse of their stored blood samples, using DNA analysis for investigation of mental illness while the subjects thought that the research was focused only on diabetes—serves as a case in point that scientific research is not free from ideology and that, given the power/resource differential between the scientists and their subject populations, there needs to be a fuller understanding of the implications of genetic data collection and usage.[34]

As noted at the outset, there are hotly contested and strongly competing explanations for differing health outcomes by ethnicity and race. In a recent paper, researchers report variable outcomes among coronary artery disease patients by ethnicity and race, and the framework that guides the empirical investigation was the deep domain assumption that biology and/or genetic differences could explain differences between population groups.[35] In this paper, the authors pay particular attention to differences between Asian populations and what they term "Western populations" (i.e., lumping together non-Asians). And even though the abstract hints that the differences are noteworthy, the content of the paper points in a different direction—namely, that the results are null regarding ethnic differences defined in the study. This leads to the question of why we have this emphasis upon racialization as biogenetic when we have strong data indicating that poverty, environmental factors, and structural relations between groups are far better candidates for approaching this matter of "health disparities."

One of the best summaries of this alternative approach now available to the general public is a seven-part series aired by the Public Broadcasting Service in 2008, which provided extensive documentation of environmental causes of disease and illness. The series was titled *Unnatural Causes: Is Inequality Making Us Sick?* Unlike Michael Moore's documentary film, *Sicko*, which focused on access to healthcare after one is sick, the PBS series turned our attention to what happens to people in different environments that cause them to become ill. In the pages that follow, we offer contributions to the emerging body of literature, which places the emphasis on the larger picture—the social and political context of the relationship between race, illness, and medicine.

NOTES

1. Nicholas Von Hoffman, "The Rich Get Thinner, The Poor Get Diabetes," *New York Observer*, http://observer.com/2006/01/the-rich-get-thinner-the-poor-get-diabetes-2/ (accessed July 26, 2012).

2. Michelle Alexander, *The New Jim Crow: Mass Incarceration in the Age of Colorblindness* (New York: The New Press, 2010).

3. Troy Duster, "The Molecular Reinscription of Race," *Patterns of Prejudice* 40, no. 4–5 (November 2006).

4. Jane DeMouy, "The Pima Indians and Genetic Research," http://diabetes.niddk.nih.gov/dm/pubs/pima/genetic/genetic.htm (accessed June 27, 2012).

5. Karl J. Reinhard et al., "Understanding the Pathoecological Relationship between Ancient Diet and Modern Diabetes through Coprolite Analysis," *Current Anthropology* 53, no. 4 (2012): 506.

6. Karen Siegel et al., "Finding a Policy Solution to India's Diabetes Epidemic," *Health Affairs* 27, no. 4 (July 2008): 1077–90.

7. H. King and M. Rewers, "Global Estimates for Prevalence of Diabetes Mellitus and Impaired Glucose Tolerance," *Diabetes Care* 16 (1993): 157–77.

8. Sandra Steingraber, *Living Downstream* (New York: Random House, 1997), 59–60.

9. Robert N. Proctor, *Cancer Wars: How Politics Shapes What We Know and Don't Know about Cancer* (New York: Basic Books, 1995), 54–74.

10. Steingraber, 61–62.

11. L. W. Pickle et al., "The New United States Cancer Atlas," *Recent Results in Cancer Research* 114 (1989): 196–207.

12. Robert D. Bullard, *Dumping in Dixie: Race, Class and Environmental Quality* (Boulder, CO: Westview Press, 1990); Julie Sze, "Gender, Asthma Politics, and Urban Environmental Justice Activism," in *New Perspectives on Environmental Justice: Gender, Sexuality, and Activism*, ed. Rachel Stein (New Brunswick, NJ: Rutgers University Press, 2004); and Julie Sze, *Noxious New York: The Racial Politics of Urban Health and Environmental Justice* (Cambridge, MA: MIT Press, 2006).

13. Produced by California Newsreel, available at http://www.unnaturalcauses.org.

14. Troy Duster, "Human Genetics and Human Taxonomies: Fluidity, Continuity and Transformations," *Transforming Racial Images: Analyses of Representations*, proceedings of the Twelfth Kyoto University International Symposium, Kyoto, Japan (2009): 81–102.

15. The HUGO Pan-Asian SNP Consortium, "Mapping Human Genetic Diversity in Asia," *Science* 11 (December 2009): 1541–45.

16. Tony S. Mok et al., "Gefitinib or Carboplatin-Paclitaxel in Pulmonary Adenocarcinoma," *New England Journal of Medicine* 361, no. 10 (2009): 947–57.

17. Jian Wang et al., "The Diploid Sequence of an Asian Individual," *Nature* 56 (November 6, 2008): 60–65.

18. Duana Fullwiley, "The Biologistical Construction of Race: 'Admixture' Technology and the New Genetic Medicine," *Social Studies of Science* 38, no. 5 (2008): 695–735; Duana Fullwiley, "The Molecularization of Race: Institutionalizing Human Difference in Pharmacogenetics Practice," *Science as Culture* 16, no. 1 (2007): 1–30; Troy Duster, "Race and Reification in Science," *Science* 307 (February 18, 2005): 1050–51; and Troy Duster, "Comparative Perspectives and Competing Explanations: Taking on the Newly Configured Reductionist Challenge to Sociology," *American Sociological Review* 71 (February 2006): 1–15.

19. Ruha Benjamin, "A Lab of Their Own: Genomic Sovereignty as Postcolonial Science Policy," *Policy and Society* 28 (2009): 341–55.

20. Ibid., 341.

21. B. Séguin et al., "Genomics, Public Health and Developing Countries: The Case of the Mexican National Institute of Genomic Medicine (INMEGEN)," *Nature Reviews Genetics* (2008): S5–S9.

22. Benjamin, 344.

23. B. Séguin et al., "Genomic Medicine and Developing Countries: Creating a Room of Their Own," *Nature Reviews Genetics* 9 (2008): 487–93.

24. Neil Risch et al., "Categorizations of Humans in Biological Research: Genes, Race and Disease," *Genome Biology* 3, no. 7 (July 1, 2002): 2007.1–2007.12; and González E. Burchard et al., "The Importance of Race and Ethnic Background in Biomedical Research and Clinical Practice," *New England Journal of Medicine* 348 (2003): 1170–75.

25. Nicholas Zamisak and Jeanne Whalen, "Cancer Drug Helps Asians Even as It Fails in Other Groups," *Wall Street Journal*, May 4, 2005.

26. Greg Gibson and G. P. Copenhaver, "Consent and Internet-Enabled Human Genomics," *PLOS Genetics* 6 (June 24, 2010), http://www.plosgenetics.org/article/info:doi/10.1371/journal.pgen.1000965 (accessed August 8, 2012).

27. Joan H. Fujimura and Ramya Rajagopalan, "Different Differences: The Use of 'Genetic Ancestry' versus Race in Biomedical Human Genetic Research," *Social Studies of Science* 41, no. 1 (2011): 5–30.

28. Benjamin, 349.

29. Mary Jane Friedrich, "Using EGFR Status to Personalize Treatment: Lung Cancer Researchers Reach a Milestone," *Journal of the National Cancer Institute* 101, no. 15 (2009): 1039–41.

30. Mok, 947–57.

31. Gang Cheng, "Clinical Review of Iressa for the Treatment of NSCLC," *Chinese Journal of Clinical Oncology* 2, no. 5 (2005): 829–33.

32. Gina Kolata, "New Treatments and Questions," *International Herald Tribune*, April 21, 2010.

33. Nantiya Tangwisutijit, "Genetic Research Raises Thorny Ethical Issues," *The Nation* (Thailand), May 1, 2005.

34. Troy Duster, "Ancestry Testing and DNA: Uses, Limits—and Caveat Emptor," in *Race and the Genetic Revolution: Science, Myth and Culture*, ed. S. Krimsky and K. Sloan (New York: Columbia University Press, 2010); and Jonathan Marks, "Science, Samples and People," *Anthropology Today* 26, no. 3 (June 2010): 3–4.

35. Jae-Sik Jang et al., "Meta-Analysis of Cytochrome P450 2C19 Polymorphism and Risk of Adverse Clinical Outcomes among Coronary Artery Disease Patients of Different Ethnic Groups Treated with *Clopidogrel*," *American Journal of Cardiology* 110, no. 4 (August 15, 2012): 502–8, http://dx.doi.org/10.1016/j.amjcard.2012.04.020 (accessed August 9, 2012).

Part II

The Personal Essay

In 1580, Michel de Montaigne published the first two volumes of his *Essais*, creating the personal essay as we know it. James Baldwin and Richard Rodriguez, among many others, continued this tradition of writing as they examined race and identity in America. The authors here, all humbled by the great prose of these thinkers, attempt to consider race and medicine with similar personal narratives. A. Pérez, for example, writes in a language and style and imagery that takes us far beneath the surface of what a Hispanic is, to describe the very people we're talking about in the medicine chapters. But is this form—rather than the traditional writing of social science or public health—useful, or even necessary?

THREE

On Meeting Richard Rodriguez

Richard Garcia

I began reading Latin American literature late. During a slow month in the neonatal ICU as an intern, I asked my friend if there were any consequential books I might read. He named three: one by a French writer, one by a Japanese writer, and *One Hundred Years of Solitude*, by a Colombian. I went to Brentano's on the west side of LA and couldn't remember any of the authors' names, or the titles of the first two books. But the Colombian's title remained in my head, with "solitude" intriguing me more than the hundred years. Naturally, when I read the book, I didn't understand it. I read more after that—Cortazar, Borges, Vargas Llosa, and the others—who all seemed headed toward the same place in antiquity: the knight errant. I then read Cervantes's big book, *Don Quixote*. About this time, perhaps like the psychotic, chivalric narrator, an ancestor of sorts, I found myself consumed by these books in my room. In a moment of clarity, I wondered whether "Mexican American" works could fit into this Latinate labyrinth at all.

I'd read books at Berkeley in Afro-American literature courses that seemed to suggest the answers to such a metaphysical trick for Black people today. That is, I could compare my own existence with a Black teenager's in Chicago who struggles to stand on the scale of humanity in a country where his humanity was rejected at the outset. A certain Bigger Thomas, then. A Mexican native son. I imagined a Mexican narrator who considers, say, the narrator of Ellison's *Invisible Man* his mentor. (His narrator, not Ellison himself.) I wrote a novel, *Conquistador's Daughter*, about some characters based on my second cousins outside of Chicago. I thought these people might give me the narratorial distance I needed as I considered my own identity as a Mexican in America who's never even been to Mexico. But the question of my existence, at all, comes from the above paragraph, and not from my second cousins' lives. For their part, they think I'm nuts.

One Hundred Years of Solitude led me into that labyrinth of Latin American literature I had not considered. Coincidently, I saw a book in the Hispanic section of the bookstore on LA's west side: *Days of Obligation: An Argument with My Mexican Father*. The title, which I didn't understand, intrigued me. I recognized the author's name: Rodriguez.

I never considered reading his first book, *Hunger of Memory: The Education of Richard Rodriguez*, while at Berkeley. I'd heard that the book trumpeted assimilation, which I rejected in those days—and since, for that matter—as a metaphysical impossibility.

I don't remember if I stood alone in the bookstore and read a paragraph or two, skipped around, and noticed some nice sentences. Or else, if I press myself, perhaps I read snatches of one of the middle chapters, "The Head of Joaquin Murrieta," and recognized a certain past. In the end, I bought *Days of Obligation* and instantly understood that it was written for me, in a way. I then bought *Hunger of Memory*, began reading it, and waited to get to the parts with which I disagreed. His style moved me. The content, too, helped me examine my own Mexicanness, which I didn't suspect I'd find interesting, and even inspired me to write on being Mexican. But I was not a writer. I didn't understand what Rodriguez did, why he wrote, or how I might follow his lead. Though he was not my leader, nor was I his follower, I thought I'd send him a letter, in any case. A letter of confession. While I didn't expect Rodriguez to write back, I didn't expect him to ignore me, either. That is, I had no expectations at all.

Richard wrote a generous letter. I've forgotten much of what he said, but do remember this line: Whether we agree on *this* or *that* isn't important. There were lines before and after this one. I wrote again. And he wrote back. We talked on the phone a few times. I was to meet Richard Rodriguez for coffee in San Francisco.

I went to his home where we chatted for a few minutes before walking down the streets of San Francisco to a coffee house where people knew him. I recall a framed print on Richard's wall: Maximilian's bloody shirt after he'd faced the Mexican firing squad.

Richard suggested that I read a few authors. I thought I'd start from the beginning, with Montaigne. I also recalled a reference to St. Augustine in Richard's piece, "Late Victorians." I read the personal narratives of essayists, collections from the past, from the present, and struggled to find what this form was. I staggered into the essays of two poets, Paz and Brodsky. They convinced me, more than the others, that this form was more than artsy prose by poets. It was a way in.

I asked myself Montaigne's question: *What do I know?*

I found a copy of a James Baldwin collection in a box of my old college books. I read it. Then bought another. And another. I'd read assigned Baldwin essays in the past, though not because they were personal essays I longed to decipher, but for their content, like a good college social science pre-medical student. I didn't recognize the personal essay, then, as craft, per se.

I called Richard and told him that I wanted to write. I don't know what I hoped he would say. Encouragement, I suppose. I talked to him like a little brother might talk to a substantial and older brother. Richard, I found through reading his essays, had grown up forty miles and twenty years from my childhood. I mean, we had central California in common. He was Mexican, like me. We had that, too. I tried to read his work to help me answer my own questions of racial, ethnic, and cultural identity. I was successful in some parts, and not in others. It turns out that Richard didn't write for me.

I said to him, "I'm from Stockton, and I don't know what I might have to say about things."

Richard replied, "Everybody's from Stockton."

The personal essayist disclosed a reality I could not have considered on my own. Then he detracted from my starry-eyed narrative and said, "You're a doctor. The noblest profession. Why do you want to write? You should be saving babies' lives." He still tells me this, although he has relented some, as I've persisted away.

I wrote some essays in those early days: grandmother, stepfather, father, childhood friends. Content and style. But no intent, really. I never thought that writing must *do* something. I still don't. But *I* wanted to do something.

My friend, a rhetorician from Berkeley, and I talked about what might make my writing good. "The story itself is the good part," he said. He urged me to work less on trying to concoct some narrative to tell someone something: "It's as if you're writing to the air. Who is your intended audience?"

This question of audience troubled me as I wrote stories about half-dead uncles, a half-dead brother, dead grandmothers, dead fathers, and, even better, a dead stepfather. None were any good, I admit here.

I went to a meeting in Chicago where the rhetorician was scheduled to chair a panel, "Apologia in American Sports," at the National Communications Association annual convention. I'd taken four sociology classes from Harry Edwards, founder of a new field, Sociology of Sport, at Berkeley, and thought that the scholarly panel would be interesting. Further, I wanted to know what happens at these academic events. I flew into O'Hare. My friend picked me up and drove me back to his house on campus. In airport traffic we managed through the usual airport greeting topics. I don't remember the details of our mindless conversation, but I started talking about race in medicine. I looked out of the window at the cars on all sides and spoke about the absurdity of race in medicine, about how all medical students learn to use "race" in the introductory part of a medical presentation—"This is a forty-year-old Hispanic," or "a three-year-old Asian," or "a fourteen-year-old African American male from South Central with a positive tox screen"—and told this professor of argument that this line of medical instruction misses the point.

I stared at the mess of cars outside.

"Richard, it sounds like you're refuting the *way* medicine is taught in America, and you don't even seem to be enthusiastic about what you're saying," he argued.

"Medical schools have been teaching this for a hundred years. This is nothing new."

"Well, it's new if you're saying that all medical schools are wrong. You should write an article about this."

It took some convincing. I honestly thought I was just making small talk in airport traffic. In the end, I wrote the essay, which was a practical transcription of what I'd said in traffic. This transcription, let's call it "The Misuse of Race in Medical Education," as much as the editors would allow, was a cleaned-up version of how I might narrate anything at all. I'd read some Montaigne and St. Augustine by then. Baldwin and Rodriguez. I don't believe I'd yet read Auden. More than these, I confess, my "natural style" (which is an impossibility, I understand) originates in that great summer between tenth and eleventh grade when I listened to the eternal eight-track of *Richard Pryor's Greatest Hits* while I slept on the summer night floor in our Stockton living room.

This is not to say that I think of my narratives as derivative (not an entirely bad word) of Richard Pryor or Richard Rodriguez. No. My speech, and, in turn, my writing, comes from an earlier time.

My "training," let's call it, begins in the sixth grade when my friends and I stopped at Grier's Liquor Store on the way home from school. We'd eat candy in the parking lot, fool around, and have a good time. We'd eventually make it home unharmed. Enriched, as it turns out. I realize now that while I look upon these days fondly, I was a twelve-year-old hanging out in a liquor store parking lot. As a pediatrician and as a parent, not to mention as a sensible person, I don't recommend hanging out in liquor store parking lots in already-dangerous neighborhoods for young children. Or anyone, for that matter. Still, if I happen to find myself in a liquor store parking lot or a medical boardroom or a scholarly conference, my early "training," it turns out, is most useful. I mean to say, no one's going to sell me a gold watch.

As a college student at Berkeley, when I taught chemistry to gifted high school students, my south Stockton ways emerged creatively and substantially. My boss had sent me to give a lecture to a group of un-achievers because of my "upbringing." As I stood on stage lecturing to them about south Stockton, Berkeley, my medical school aspirations, and their potential lives, I had another one of my epiphanies. My boss had asked me to inspire these high school unachievers. What else could I do? I told them about my uncle in prison; my other recently dead uncle's heroin miscalculation; my father, whom I'd only met three or four times, sitting in a liquor store parking lot in the years before his own heroin overdose; and the rest. While on stage explaining how my life had emerged without even my own expectation, I realized that my boss said she'd pay me my regular chemistry-tutoring rate of $10 an hour, but did not specify the denominator. So, if I talked for two hours, I'd make $20. It's a deal! I spoke to these unachievers for two hours, prepared only with what I brought with me that day: my personal narrative.

* * *

Many years later I sat in the audience at the National Medical Association Scientific Convention as Surgeon General David Satcher, MD, PhD, spoke. The topic was "health disparities." I'd not yet heard that term. As I sat through his speech, I realized what was missing from my own keynote speech earlier that year at a university conference on cultural competence. The director of the conference invited me to give the keynote after reading my article taken from the Chicago traffic jam. I gave the same speech I'd given in Oakland the month before. However, the new audience and I endured a great distance. I didn't understand how these same words could succeed in Oakland, yet fail at this university. Among the other obvious reasons, I now suspect that I had not yet considered disparities in health based on race, and could not assemble my words into an academic context for this audience. At the very least, some mention of this distinction would have located my words on race and medicine such that the audience could make more sense of what I was up to in my speech. But I wasn't up to a speech on disparities, it turns out. It wasn't until I heard Dr. Satcher that I was able to link my traffic jam article to a tangible, deadly issue and relieve it of its mere observation of race in a superficial American medical education.

I wrote more articles on race and medicine. I argued for interdisciplinarity and tangibility. I gave speeches, talked on the phone with friends, taught medical students and residents in patients' rooms. And here's this book.

My friend, Troy Duster, a great sociologist, and I talked on the phone. I asked him how someone can become an expert on race. Troy quipped, "It's like instant coffee. You just add hot water, and *voilà!*"

I thought I should also read more. I read what I could find in the standard medical journals, the 2002 Institute of Medicine report titled *Unequal Treatment*, and the other standard pieces. I became increasingly bothered by health disparities as an uncontroverted mainstay in my profession, my country. I conceived this book. But how could I write it? And to what end?

I thought about how a piece on race and medicine would be different, in my hands, than the other standard pieces on the shelves. In the end, I didn't think physicians, ourselves, would be able to cure chronic health disparities in America. I thought I should get some coauthors with wide collective expertise to write this book of personal narratives. Not as gimmick, but as synecdoche, the way I've thought since those early after-noons at Grier's Liquor Store and beyond.

But what would be my intent?

In general, when I discuss the idea of a book on health disparities, people want to know what the solutions will be. Like a recipe for oatmeal cookies, where they can turn to the section on solutions and apply those to stamp out disparities wherever they are, culminating in a batch of soft cookies with nuts, perhaps. But when I say I'm interested in locating the discussion on race and medicine differently than it currently exists, I'm easily dismissed. However, such dismissals have never bothered me. When Baldwin wrote about race in America, he went back to Paris and didn't solve anything at all on the racial front. I don't mean to compare myself to Baldwin, of course. Rather, I mean to invite our attention to a crushing human existence.

Each time I read an article about, say, a Mexican in pain not getting pain medication at the same dose and with the same quickness as his White counterpart, I wonder how long I'd have to sit in pain. I'm a doctor. Would that get me anywhere? When my wife was in pain in the ER, was the delay in treating her pain related to her being Black? To the doctor's being White? To something not entirely neat that could fit in a medical essay?

Yes, I suspect.

What could I do? If I were to demand that she be evaluated by the doctor now, and given narcotics now, I would only have been seen by the outside world as an agitated Mexican in the ER asking for narcotics. By "outside world," I suppose I mean the security guard.

Eventually, the nurse took my wife into a room, the doctor came in, examined her, and said he'd order some pain medication and call the obstetrician. I asked him which medication he planned to order. The ER doctor walked right up to my face and aggressively asked what I thought he should order.

As a tall, threatening, Mexican man, none of which are my fault, I looked down upon the ER doctor and said, "I want her to have what's best. Now."

Medicine is not the big picture, but the little one. Further examination of race in America seems necessary for better concrete medical results, if we are interested. It's this "we" that remains in question, I worry. Every-one can say, "Sure, count me in. Let's do better for racial minorities. Let's improve their health status, give [or sell, I should say] them better care, and be a better country. Better people." This makes financial sense. And moral sense.

Of course, physicians can't do this on their own. Not in medical practice, and not in medical education. Because this is not a medical complication that will be solved among doctors, if at all. Rather, this is an American complication, for those interested, requiring scholars from all around to ultimately bring us to a *deliberative* discourse, in fact. Anything less promises to be anemic, no matter how forceful.

From Michel de Montaigne and St. Augustine and James Baldwin and Richard Rodriguez emerged a form I could attempt as I considered particular episodes in my life as they bespeak the tenets of health disparities. I'm no saint. No medieval thinker. Nor do I follow the lines of Baldwin or Rodriguez. Rather, I sit around and ask myself, as often as I can stand it, *What do I know?* And then I attempt to write an answer that might help my mother, a sixty-four-year-old Mexican woman with asthma who visited her physician, a new medical school graduate working in a hospital where poor, underinsured, and uninsured patients go for healthcare. The young doctor abruptly discontinued my mother's asthma medications. As I drove with her on a Sunday evening, she could only say two or three words without gasping for air. I called the young doctor assigned to her care, who happened to be working that Sunday, and asked why he'd stopped her asthma medications. He said, "I remember your mother. She doesn't have asthma. She passed the test."

To which I replied, "There is no test for asthma. It's a clinical diagnosis. Further, she 'passed the asthma test' when she was on her asthma medications."

My mother, born in Stockton, like her mother, speaks English and works as a housekeeper, when she can. She's not yet old enough to receive Medicare benefits. She is uninsured. And she is sick. Because I'm a physician, I was able to call a pharmacy to prescribe her medications that Sunday night. This kept her breathing until she could see her young doctor two days later. Her alternative was to sit in a hospital ER and wait, without insurance, or time, on her side. (Let's admit, it is unusual for a poor Mexican woman to ride around on Sundays with a doctor for a son.)

Or else I could offer my brother, who lives as if he were living in the pre-antibiotic era, draining pus from his shoulder with pressure and hot-as-he-could-stand boiled towels because this was the best he could do, as an example of the sort of healthcare people can expect to receive. Since I'm a pediatrician, I really shouldn't be treating my adult family's asthma, diabetes, and abscesses.

Someone else should.

Health disparities exist between races in America. Hundreds of studies, reports, conferences, articles, and seminars catalog them. The proposed solutions to eliminating, or at least decreasing, these eternal disparities are apparently insufficient to close the gap between the races. The mainstays of proposed solutions—cultural and linguistic competence, medical student and physician diversity, health insurance, access to care, electronic health records, and so forth—are promoted as the very tools necessary to close the gap in both health *status* and health *care*, even as they fail. Of course, these items are necessary, in part, as our country continues its insistence on race. More studies cataloging racial differences in healthcare would be superfluous.

Yet practical solutions to these disparities remain anemic.

A Black man with chest pain waits longer than a White man for his initial EKG. The answer is to step on it, kick it into high gear, pick up the pace, get the EKG done, interpret it correctly, and treat the patient right. Every time.

A Black or Mexican man with a long bone fracture in the emergency room waits longer for a smaller dose of pain medication when compared with a fractured White leg. The answer is to get these men in pain the correct dose of morphine.

Stat.

Certainly, thousands of doctors treat Black or Mexican patients with high-quality care. These people are in the best hands and will suffer no disparities as cataloged over the last couple of centuries. But disparities, when looking at populations of patients, comprised of individuals—people, then—happen because a physician or a nurse or a healthcare "system" fails to administer the right treatment for racial minorities with the same "quality," let's call it, as for Whites. And if they do experience disparate care in a crowded, poor clinic or ER, then we can say it's a matter of money, or some other pesky insurance or income practicality. This would be simple. Nevertheless, if a brown person with a stroke happens to live near a stroke center, then she's likely to get the standard national treatment with respect to time. If she doesn't, as so many don't, then she's out of luck.

But this is not just luck in question. Disparities are not haphazard coincidences.

The location at which the Mexican man shows up with slurred speech matters. It's better to have a stroke in Palo Alto than at my mother's apartment. When we're looking at how to decrease disparities across a population of racial minority countrymen and women, finding a translator for me won't work, as I only speak English; arguing for increased insurance access for Kaiser members won't work, as they all have Kaiser cards; standardized algorithms for Spanish-speaking Mexicans with chest pain who clutch their chests in pain far from a Center of Excellence won't work; completing a cultural competence course where the physician learns not to touch a Thai kid on the head won't work.

But if we develop a rhetorical environment in which this complexity can be appreciated, made particular, applied, monitored, rewarded, and enforced, we will have directed the audience in a better direction toward solutions. I suppose I am pessimistic, by all accounts. Can we make the case to decrease health disparities on financial grounds? On pathetic grounds? On a combination of grounds that is nimble enough to apply differentially when apt?

Who will be the audience for this persuasive speech?

Describing health disparities is a job already well done. What we *do* about them, and, more to the point, *how* we persuade anyone to do anything about them, is some of what's at stake.

Race and healthcare equality have been in question since America's beginning: through the early, infant years; during the Civil War and Reconstruction; when hospitals were born and then evolved, through the Flexnor Report, and the discovery of penicillin; at the forcible integration of hospitals, in the 1960s, and at the invention of the CT scan and the MRI, during the pharmaceutical flourishing, burgeoning Medicaid, Medicare, and HMOs, two Puerto Rican surgeons general, three Black surgeons general, and a Kenyan American president.

No arc currently exists as we examine the ultimate goal: end health disparities, which, as Troy Duster points out, isn't quite the same as improving the health of people at the bottom. *How* we arrive at healthcare in the United States that is appropriate for everyone, race notwithstanding, remains a bitter question. And by "we," I suppose I'm talking about us all.

I'm not talking about equality here. If I have two patients in the ER waiting for me to treat them—one in respiratory distress and the other with a diaper rash—equality is not the best approach. If I treated them equally, one baby would receive a fantastic diaper cream, or the other wouldn't survive. Rather, each should receive the appropriate care for his or her medical condition.

The answer to health disparities in the United States remains hidden. On the one hand, it's quite simple: provide high-quality care to everyone at all times. When I think about the complexity of our history and of our social present, I cannot imagine a cleaner, more practical, less attainable solution. I'm reminded of a question posed to then Senator Obama about a city ordinance, I think it was, being considered to force young men to wear their pants at their waists, and not far below. Senator Obama said something like "We don't need a policy. Brothers just need to pull up their pants."

I sometimes work in a busy pediatric office where I see exclusively poor Mexicans—from either Mexico or California. Most speak only Spanish. Ten exam rooms, two or three pediatricians, one or two nurse practitioners.

A grandmother brought her seventeen-year-old grandson in for a routine adolescent exam at nine in the morning. "Doctor, I'm worried because he's abusing alcohol," she said.

I replied in general, "He's too young to drink."

"Tell him, Doctor! Tell him! I'm worried, too, because his mother has hepatitis C. She's a heroin addict. His father is also an addict. Heroin, and other drugs. Even my husband is dying because of heroin. Me? I've never done drugs in my life. But I'm worried about my grandson. Do you think it has something to do with the environment? I don't want this life for him."

Nine a.m. I wasn't ready to hear such a story. This neighborhood office is near a small community hospital. A gas station on the corner. A taco stand across the street. The small pharmacy on the other corner reminds me of the one near my childhood pediatrician's office, where I'd get cherry cough drops after seeing him in 1970s Stockton.

Nor was I ready to step into the role of *doctor* for this *kind* of patient in this *kind* of clinic—first thing. I typically examine about fifty-five patients per eight-hour day there: vaccines, gastroenteritis, wheezing, conjunctivitis, ear infections, simple viral colds, antibiotics versus nasal suction discussions with parents, formula switching, WIC forms, school notes. Fifty-five patients each day. My days there are mostly in Spanish, which is not my language.

But the culture is definitely mine.

Both the grandmother and the grandson spoke English, like my grandmother and I spoke to each other before she died when I was in the sixth grade. While I decline to accept that this boy's family life surrounded by drugs is cultural, in a broad sense, I could not help but recognize my own past in the narrative of his present.

I looked right inside the seventeen-year-old and said something along the lines of my old speeches during my college chemistry job: My Uncle Monchie overdosed on heroin and died when I was in college. My genetic father, whom I only met three or four times, overdosed on heroin and died when I was training in pediatrics. And my Uncle Junior overdosed on heroin and died three Christmas Eves ago.

I was born to a single mother in nineteen-sixty something. My genetic father had no tangible effect on my life, which was good for me, it turns out. My grandfather, all of his brothers, all of my uncles, and all of my male cousins went to prison. Thieves, primarily.

The adolescent boy looked back into me. Either my imagination or my clinical pride construed his look as evidence of the *kind* of medicine I thought I'd practice when I chose to become a pediatrician during my own adolescence, when I was about his age. Or else my imagination failed me and I made no greater doctor-patient connection than anyone else might have, or any more than I might have by simply counseling a parent about ear infections and the overuse of antibiotics. I don't know if I directed him toward a better life with words, medical treatment, and referrals. Maybe I did. I won't ever know.

Where people receive healthcare certainly matters. But this has little to do with actual geography—a meridian, a latitude, building construction, proximity to houses or bus lines, side of town. More than these items, the location in question has to do with the *product quality* that racial minority people can expect to receive when they seek healthcare, wherever they find it.

The seventeen-year-old drinking alcohol interests me. It's not an exaggeration to say that *he is the reason* I became a doctor.

His height and weight were normal. He had some moderate acne on his face, sparing his chest, back, and shoulders. His vision and hearing were normal. In general, he was in good overall health—except for the acne, the alcohol, and the life.

If I were working in a university or county hospital or integrated system of healthcare, I would have had more tools available to take care of this teenager. If I, his doctor, am a variable, then I'm a constant, and the location where I saw him is the variable. While I recognize this is not real science, it'll do for now, since now is where the teenager finds himself.

I don't mean to indict doctors, physician assistants, or nurse practitioners who work in these underserved areas. The contrary is true: These healthcare deliverers—the so-called safety net—are critical in offering access to healthcare for so many people in these otherwise medically naked areas.

But they are not enough. Safety nets, as I understand them, are good for people who walk a tightrope high above a solid ground that would kill them with even the slightest misstep. I don't imagine this inspires anyone who finds himself receiving his healthcare on a tightrope he didn't know he was walking.

Health disparities require a deliberative category of speech: Close the deal. Eliminate disparities. Or, at least, bend in that direction. But ending disparities cannot be done successfully without first collecting prevailing thoughts, examining proposed solutions, broadening our possibilities, articulating the reasons (which are neither clear nor agreed upon), and, most critically, identifying the intended audience—doctors, insurance executives, politicians, medical educators, social science and health educators, patients—and concretizing their own benefits.

Money, percentage of GDP, medical quality vis-à-vis the cost we pay in the United States are necessary elements of persuading the audience that practical, tangible results benefit us all, for we all pay to take care of the ER patient with advanced disease and no insurance.

To wit, discussions about disparities require us to be nimble in our approach. The Cantonese woman needs a translator. The Ukrainian woman, too. Others need geographical access to good primary care doctors and at least reasonable geographical or financial access to good specialty care. This is not quite an issue in Westwood or Santa Monica, California, like it is for rural or poorly insured patients.

Highlighting these well-documented, but unrealized, solutions betrays the rhetorical intent of any doctor interested in healthy patients. Humanity itself is at stake. The reasons to arrive at practical solutions and change from a certain stability in disparities discourse cannot simply be financial rewards to physicians, insurance company shareholders, and taxpayers. Because we are talking about grandmothers and fathers and brothers and daughters, we can conclude, in a way, with a line from Toni Morrison's novel, *Beloved*: "This is flesh I'm talking about here."

FOUR

Geography of the Dead

A. Pérez

There is a running joke in my family, a web of stories now a part of family lore created mostly by my father. His older brother Walker (real name Joaquín) has an obsession with cleanliness. Dirt has been the bane of his life since he was a kid growing up Mexican in an immigrant farm worker village on a citrus ranch in Southern California. His family members were laborers who picked fruit for a living. They worked in the dirt. They tilled and watered it, walked in it to tend trees, and spent most of their working days in some way in or around it. Rather than living in the tidy, clean, White community in town, they lived in the "Mexican village," a workers' camp hidden behind a bank of eucalyptus trees located off a two-lane highway five miles outside of town, where there were no paved roads and where the two hundred or so 1920s shotgun houses, with no heat, served as temporary shelters for migrant farm workers. The Mexican village was, to the folks in town, a place associated with poverty, filth, and disease, the common stigma that Mexicans in that era collectively carried, as if imprinted on their backs. To this day, Uncle Walker hates almost everything about his childhood home, the Mexican village— which was demolished twenty years ago—but especially what he remembers as the inescapable plague of dirt that, we all like to say today, he's been trying to clean off of himself ever since he left the village to join the Marines at the age of eighteen.

Since then, Uncle Walker's been remarkably successful in his efforts at evading the bane of dirt. A few examples come to mind. He takes tremendous pride in his grooming, to the point of obsession. Since leaving the ranch, we like to say, his fingernails have never seen a smidgen of dirt. To impersonate him, one merely has to look at one's fingernails and check for dirt. With this simple gesture, we've always gotten a good laugh at Walker's expense. To this day, he also dresses impeccably. He avoids any clothes that might appear working class. I have never seen him in denim blue jeans. (This is what he wore on the ranch, where his family could afford only two pairs of Levi's a year for their three sons. The pants got dirty and dingy pretty fast.) As a child, I already began to notice the pattern. Today, Walker's standard attire—he prefers light-colored garments, sometimes pastels, always pressed and spotless—might be described as a hybrid of J. Crew and Banana Republic. He invented this fashion statement decades ago: deck shoes, as if he'd spent time on a yacht; casual slacks, but not brown khaki, since they might appear working class; some type of polo shirt, preferably with horizontal stripes.

When I was a kid, Uncle Walker bought a boat, which he used to take us for rides. The boat, too, seemed to conform to his dress code, or, to put it differently, my uncle dressed like a sailor or yachtsman and therefore needed a boat to seal the deal. Once, as we were docking after an afternoon of fishing, Walker was telling us kids how to properly tie up a boat. As we watched, he fell into the sooty water up to his armpits. We screamed with laughter. It was the only time I ever saw Uncle Walker with soiled clothes. Today, as if to make up for that moment of ignominy, Walker lives in a pricey area where most of the houses have a beachfront view. His house has a dock, though he sold his boat a long time ago and I doubt he ever goes near the water. He rents his dock to his neighbor, who owns a boat much bigger than Walker's was.

Walker's house on the water is so bereft of dust and germs, so unimaginably immaculate, I have little doubt that, if need be, a surgeon could use it in an emergency to perform an operation. Let's begin with the bathrooms, the place in the house where, as we all have long known, Walker has a special compunction for hygiene. Even as a child, I noticed that I'd never seen a piece of trash in any of the bathroom bins in Walker's house. Not a single balled-up tissue, a spent cardboard toilet paper tube, or even a smudge of toothpaste from a dispensed container. Like a vacuum toilet on an airliner, the bathroom waste bins in Walker's house seemed to empty themselves automatically, and the bins were kept sparkling clean. Though it seemed absurd at the time, we came to believe that Walker or his wife must have checked the bathroom and bins immediately after a guest visited the commode, which meant, of course, that while we were at Walker's house someone was "on watch," so to speak. That person mysteriously emptied the trash and tidied up after each guest.

Today the rest of Walker's house, as well as the patio and yards, measures up to the bathroom: the carpeting always recently vacuumed, the kitchen countertops freshly polished, the window glass impossibly transparent. Outside, the landscaping is maintained with a similar nod to Martha Stewart. Though raised on a ranch in "el campo," where lemon and orange orchards surrounded the Mexican village, Walker's yard shows little evidence of his family's ancestral knowledge of plants and trees, especially fruit trees. Though orange and lemon trees blossomed in my own family's yard when I was growing up, Walker never planted reminders of his life in the Mexican village.

In winter, which Uncle Walker seems to prefer because it is a time of the year that does not induce sweat, he might wear a starched and pressed dress shirt under a V-neck designer sweater or, if it's cold, a heavy Dr. Heathcliff Huxtable sweater with an argyle design. It goes without saying that, except for the sailing episode, to this day I have never seen an unholy spot on Uncle Walker's clothing or shoes. Ever.

We'd come to believe that Walker had internalized the long-held perception in the United States that Mexicans are dirty, unhygienic, and therefore wont to spread contagion and disease, or simply that they are somehow innately different from White Americans and that difference explained their "unclean habits." Clearly, we thought that Uncle Walker's obsession with cleanliness and hygiene, his punctilious evasion of dirt, stemmed from the shame that was driven into him growing up poor and Mexican during a time when Mexicans had little opportunity to resist or rebut the stereotype. In that era, such hateful sentiments toward Mexicans served to justify Jim Crow segregation, of which Walker and his family had been victims.

Our bemused fascination with Walker's obsession over the years derived from a collection of stories about Walker's childhood, as told by my father. Because their elder sister Miranda had excelled in the segregated Mexican (American) elementary school in the Mexican village, she, and

later her brothers, were permitted to attend the local White schools—
a privilege granted to only a handful of the Mexican kids. If one child in
the family was smart, the others probably were as well, teachers assumed, an assumption my father liked to say he disproved. Aunt Miranda would later become a psychiatric nurse and marry a psychiatrist. She
eventually became a therapist herself, and currently treats primarily Latino immigrant clients. Walker, now retired, worked in the quality control
department for the McDonnell Douglas Corp.

The privilege of attending the White schools had its "challenges" for
Walker and his brothers. They'd been isolated from the White community and were therefore not accustomed to the world outside the village's
comfort zone. They now faced the full brunt of Jim Crow–era racism for
the first time, a hatred that was all the more brutal given that it occurred
in a school setting, where they expected to be protected. White kids,
echoing what they heard in their homes or saw in the movies of that era,
called Walker and his brothers "dirty Mexicans," among other things.
"Dirty," like today, seemed a favorite term of opprobrium to level at
Mexicans. After all, their status as farm workers proved Mexicans were
dirty, as did their "swarthy oily skin." "Some of them were as black as
Negros! And they ate mostly beans and tortillas, not bread. And look
where they lived!"

Mexican mothers in the village would awaken early each morning to
prepare food for their families, including lunches for the kids. Like most
of the other kids, Walker and his siblings left for school each morning
with bags of carefully wrapped burritos. These were made from homemade flour tortillas, rolled from fresh dough and cooked on a *comal* in the
morning darkness by Walker's mother. This was arduous work, especially when making lunches for five kids and one's husband. Each tortilla
enveloped a helping of pinto beans, probably refried because this added
flavor, cooked in a large pot with bacon and garlic on the small gas stove
(also used for heating) in the tiny kitchen.

An overview of the village's geography: The workers' camp was built
along the north bank of the Sespe River, in that day the last free-flowing
river in Southern California. When the kids left to catch the bus each
morning, they walked away from the river toward the state highway,
perhaps a fifteen-minute walk. Of the two dirt roads into the village, one
followed another smaller river that flowed from the San Cayetano Mountains into the bigger one below. The kids took this road to get to school.

The walk was usually uneventful, except for my father, who remembered something that never left him, even when he grew old and feeble and had already forgiven Walker for everything from childhood and after.

Along the way to the bus stop each morning, Walker regularly tossed his mother's burritos, his only source of nourishment for the day, into the river before the bus arrived. To avoid eating Mexican food in front of the White kids at school, he jettisoned, like unnecessary ballast, his lunch burritos every day. Walker would rather go hungry than be seen eating food that would identify him as Mexican. My father would re-create this scene in good humor at family events to remind Walker of his early "transgressions." In these stories the burritos became explosive "hand grenades" that pockmarked the river, thrown with the precision of a combat veteran at an imaginary foe. Walker would laugh uneasily and shrug it off.

But the metaphor was not far off the mark. My father had no problem consuming burritos in front of the White kids at school. Once he'd even imagined ways of retrieving and salvaging the lost aluminum foil–sealed nuggets from the river. For him the burritos were "grenades" of a sort, because under the Jim Crow regime the mere act of eating them at the White school was a symbolic statement of pride that flew in the face of anti-Mexican sentiment. For my father, Mexican culture meant nourishment and strength, not something to be hidden or jettisoned out of shame, as if such a thing were possible. Unlike Walker, he embraced the stigma stamped on his back as an act of defiance, knowing full well that such stereotypes were racist myths. My psychiatrist uncle, an Irish American who was close to our family and would become a sort of honorary Chicano, once remarked on the fundamental difference between Walker and my father. Some time back, when they were both young, he told my father, "The difference between you and Walker is that he hates being Mexican while you love it."

Walker's obsession with cleanliness could not be viewed as a mere idiosyncratic habit, nor could it be reduced to, or explained solely by, his relationship to his ethnic background. Rather, it was certainly part eccentricity, one of those odd habits that anyone might possess no matter what his cultural background, akin to the kind of obsessive miserliness that fiction writers have captured in a number of memorable characters — Dickens's Ebenezer Scrooge, Molière's Harpagon, or Faulkner's Jason Compson. But Walker's scrupulous hygiene and related habits were also in part—perhaps in large part—a complex psychological defense mechanism that allowed him to keep at bay some of the demons he'd long felt compelled to repress.

In college I couldn't help but recall other characters in literature who shared Uncle Walker's habit. Obsessive hand washing, for example, seemed to be a favorite device in Shakespeare's plays. Lady Macbeth, who conspired with her husband to murder King Duncan, washes her hands for a quarter of an hour; Macbeth does the same, saying that even the ocean couldn't wash his hands clean of Duncan's blood. Claudius, who usurped the throne by murdering his brother, Hamlet's father, says that there isn't enough rain in the heavens to wash his hands clean of his brother's blood. Freud, who drew from classic literature, identified obsessive hand washing as an unconscious activity that resulted from a neurosis originating in guilt and/or anxiety.

Though Walker certainly hadn't committed any crime, could his inordinate cleanliness have something to do with his childhood experiences as a Mexican living under Jim Crow? Or did the idiosyncratic habit stem from his guilt over having repressed the racial demons of his past? Was it, as Freud might have posited, an unconscious expression of guilt, perhaps for having "killed" his other (Mexican) self? There was no evading one fact: Foremost among the demons that Walker and other Mexican Americans who came of age during the Jim Crow era faced was the ghostly presence of their Mexican alter ego, their very cultural identity as children of Mexican immigrants (in Walker's case, his very sense of *being* as a native son of the Mexican village).

When Walker was growing up, every facet of life in town was segregated, including housing, schools, movie theaters, and barber shops. Since there were no Blacks in town, Jim Crow targeted Mexicans, regardless of whether they had been born in the United States. Though Walker has never (not once) spoken about this dark side of his childhood and youth, my father told many stories about life under Jim Crow. His most memorable were his stories about segregation in the small movie theater in town. Though the theater's maximum capacity was, perhaps, 150 people, Mexicans were not allowed in the "Whites Only" section. This was not the Old South after Reconstruction, but Southern California in the 1930s and 1940s—Hollywood's Golden Era—a scenic forty-five-minute drive from downtown Los Angeles.

Decades later, when an earthquake badly damaged the theater, my Great Uncle Isidro, who still lives around the corner from the old theater, told a lady asking for donations to repair the "historic" cinema to "go to hell." Not only did Isidro not mourn the theater's near implosion from the quake, but today, at the age of eighty-nine, his blood still boils when he's asked about this episode from the town's past. My grandfather Arcadio once told me that the theater was a "flea-infested hole in the wall" anyway, compared to the theaters he'd seen as a child in the city of Zacatecas, Mexico, where today the Teatro Calderón, a nineteenth-century opera house, still stands in the old colonial downtown district. Not only were Mexicans the equal of the White Americans, my grandfather said, but they were in many ways culturally superior to them.

Another Jim Crow story was the segregated cemetery, where today, if one is familiar with the geography of the dead, one can find the old Mexican section, originally placed at the very back of the grounds. The entrance and front area hold the prominent headstones of the town's White ancestors, the "marble orchard," as Steinbeck once described them. The plaques of the town's Mexican ancestors are in the background, in what is now the middle section of the cemetery. Many Mexican American soldiers who died in World War II, Korea, and Vietnam—some of whom were my father's school friends—were buried here. Joe Salazar was one. He and my father used to go hunting for rabbits in the local hills. My father said Joe was the best shot he'd ever seen. An old photo with a couple dozen rabbits lined up was the proof. Like all of his friends from the Mexican village, including my father, at the age of eighteen, Joe had volunteered for the army at the start of the Korean War. He was killed three months after arriving in Korea, but his body wasn't found for another six months. One day my father and I were walking through the cemetery reading the names on the plaques. We stumbled across Joe Salazar's grave. This was only the second time I ever saw my father cry.

At the core of Jim Crow segregation was the assumption that Blacks and other "colored" people in the United States posed a safety and/or health threat and must therefore be kept away from Whites. The underlying rationale for the segregation of Blacks was that, given that they were deemed to be "animalistic," they (especially men) were believed to be sexually incontinent, or unable to control their sex drive. This meant that if Black men were permitted near White women, mass rape would be the outcome. Jim Crow in the Southwest differed in many ways from that of other regions of the country; there were also different localized versions throughout the South and the rest of the United States, though the basic racial logic remained the same.

When I teach Mexican American literature and history, I am disturbed by the level of ignorance among students of Jim Crow segregation in the Southwest. Many students believe that such racism occurred only in the South. In the Southwest, the stigma and stereotypes were also applied to Mexicans and other racial groups. The purported health threat followed from the belief that Mexicans were unclean or unhygienic and therefore wont to carry diseases. More troubling is the media-driven revival of this hurtful stereotype. Lou Dobbs, for example, raised the specter of Mexican-borne disease, specifically leprosy, in his now canceled CNN evening anti-immigrant polemic. This chilling stereotype, innocuously called *Lou Dobbs Tonight*, continues to appear in different guises on television and other electronic media. The episode, as popularized on Dobbs's show, would make for a fitting entry in an updated version of Charles Mackay's nineteenth-century book, *Extraordinary Popular Delusions and the Madness of Crowds*.

Dobbs claimed that illegal immigrants were to blame for a recent spike in leprosy cases in the United States. Did it matter that federal data dispute his assertion that there has been a recent surge in leprosy cases? The National Hansen's Disease Program, a unit of the US Department of Health and Human Services, has been collecting reports from healthcare providers and agencies in its registry since 1894. According to this office, there hasn't been a spike in leprosy cases in recent years, a period that, if critics of undocumented immigration are correct, would have provided ample proof of a correlation. Dobbs was not alone in sensationalizing the leprosy story as part of the broader argument that undocumented immigrants pose health risks to the US public; similar fear-mongering can be found on Fox News and other national news sources.

Though Jim Crow customs in the town where Walker and his family lived seemed to have disappeared by the 1970s, the legacy remains. The town is still segregated along racial lines, though not as rigidly as before, and Mexican immigrant farm workers still form the labor force on the ranches, which today are owned by the descendants of the ranchers for whom my father and his brothers worked. Those ranchers continue to be dependent on cheap Mexican and Latino labor, just as their ancestors were one hundred years ago. History repeats itself, Faulkner said. There is no such thing as "was."

My father wanted to be buried in his hometown next to his mother and father, so when he passed away in 2010 we had to make plans for a funeral there. When my brother called the only mortuary in the town, the attendant wanted to know where we were from. She didn't know that we lived in the city more than sixty miles away. By the attendant's insistence, my brother knew she wanted to know if we were from the White (upper-class) side of town or the Mexican (lower-class) side. This single phone call so infuriated my brother that when we went to the mortuary, he unleashed a few unkind words on the attendant, a short portly woman with a sad face.

My brother tried to smooth things over, but afterward he was still angry. I explained to him that we were back in rural America, and that the woman he quarreled with was an ignorant hick. But as soon as I'd met the attendant, I knew my brother was right. Though we all speak perfect English, and my brother in fact doesn't speak a word of Spanish, the attendant had assigned us to a young Spanish-speaking aide for the appointment. Was this her way of getting the last word? "Mexican" still meant that you speak Spanish and pick lemons for a living. My mother thought we'd made too much of this incident, and maybe she was right. But to this day in the town, there is no evading one fact: The word "Mexican" continues to carry a stigma—the Mark of M, if you will, a skewed version of the Mark of Zorro or the Scarlet Letter.

I imagine that Uncle Walker's worst nightmare would be a surprise Sunday morning visit to his beachfront home by a long-lost Mexican relative bearing a pot of steaming *menudo* (red chile stew). The mysterious visitor, dark-skinned, dressed like a Mexican *campesino* (peasant), in *huaraches* (sandals), and bearing the traditional stew of the poor, is, I believe, how the Devil himself would have appeared to Walker. In Walker's nightmare, this ghost of the Mexican past appears to take him back to the Mexican village. No one can see him on the porch except Walker. The Mexican offers Walker the *menudo*; when Walker lifts the lid, the stew is boiling. Walker looks at the tripe and hominy roiling in the red stew. The *campesino* says to look closer into the pot.

When Walker does, he sees that the tripe is not tripe at all, but tiny living creatures struggling in the stew, and when he looks closer he clearly distinguishes miniature human figures with their arms flailing about as they try to keep themselves above the liquid so as not to drown. Before he can see their faces, they are drawn back below the surface by the boiling currents. Walker recoils in fright and then notices that the *campesino* is holding the pot firmly with both hands, but without mittens. The Mexican says to Walker, in Spanish, "Have a bowl, my son, it's delicious."

Walker screams and wakes up. He remembers that he hasn't had a bowl of *menudo* in years, maybe decades. He considers it unclean and unhealthful, and frankly one of those things he associates with the Mexican village. You could say the Mexican stew itself represented all that Uncle Walker had sought to evade and transcend in life. *Menudo* (meaning "small pieces" of meat) is the quintessential food of the poor, made from the leftovers of the old hacienda kitchens in colonial Mexico—the intestines of farm animals, unused corn, pig's feet—but transformed by the resourcefulness of the poor into a hearty breakfast dish that today is eaten anywhere you find Mexicans.

My father embraced the term "Chicano" from a very young age. But this word, popularized in the 1960s, seemed to be anathema to Walker, or so I always assumed, since he never used it. The origins of the term explain why it still carries a lower-class connotation for many Mexicans and Mexican Americans, and also perhaps for Walker. Like most folk or slang terms, the word's derivation isn't easy to pin down. Scholars agree that "Chicano" was originally an in-group term of derision used by Mexican immigrants toward recent arrivals of largely indigenous ancestry who spoke heavily accented Spanish, their native tongue. One theory is that the dark-skinned, indigenous "Indian" Mexicans, themselves the objects of racism in Mexico, mispronounced the term "Mexicano," which rankled the nationalistic immigrants. Rather than the Mexican Spanish pronunciation, the Indians were heard speaking a dialect version, "Me-shee-cano" or "Me-chee-cano." Hence, "Chee-ca-no," or simply Chicano, became synonymous with uncouth, uneducated, and lower-class Mexican Indians. Originally, being branded "Chicano" probably meant that you were a member of the lowest group among Mexican immigrants. It was one of the folk ingredients of Mexico's linguistic *menudo*—beginning as an undesirable leftover, the tripe of the animal—until it would be adopted in the 1960s by many Mexican Americans as a symbolic term of racial and cultural pride signifying identification with their much despised and stigmatized community as well as with their bicultural identity. Although associated today with the 1960s Mexican American civil rights movement, the word Chicano in fact emerged from the Mexican barrios, workers' camps, and immigrant communities of the early 1900s.

Chicano nationalists of the 1960s would not have held my Uncle Walker in high esteem, nor would Chicano movement holdouts, who today wield the term to judge Mexican Americans who appear to them too "Anglicized" or "agringado." (This, of course, would include almost every professional or even well-educated Mexican American.) Reminiscent of Black nationalism as espoused by figures like Malcolm X, the theory goes like this: Uncle Walker suffers from a psychological malady common to many people of color of his generation, an insidious self-hatred—that is, an internalization of the hatred meted out to him as a child living under Jim Crow. Just as Walker's farm worker community was exploited and oppressed by US agri-business, Walker's mind, too, has been colonized by White America.

But could one expect my Uncle Walker to "decolonize" his mind and undergo the type of "psychic conversion" embraced by Chicano and Black nationalists alike in the 1960s? Malcolm X, whose ideas shaped all ethnic American nationalism of that decade, called for this type of "decolonization" of the mind. According to Cornel West, Malcolm X's notion of psychic conversion held that Black people should no longer view themselves through White lenses. Malcolm X claimed that Black people would never value themselves as long as they subscribed to a standard of valuation that devalued them. Their "conversion" would involve the "decolonization" of the mind that would strip White cultural standards (White supremacy) of their authority, legitimacy, and efficacy. It would begin with a bold and defiant rejection of Black degradation, and would be sustained by efforts to expand spaces wherein Black humanity is affirmed.

As West sees it, this radical transformation of the mind was less a statement against White America than an expression of love for the Black community. Transposed to the Mexican American Southwest, conversion and decolonization were embraced by Chicano nationalists as they confronted a similar legacy of Jim Crow racism. Like Malcolm X, Chicano nationalists believed that only when Mexican Americans learned to love themselves, by shedding the internalized legacy of past racism, could they truly empower themselves.

Contemporary "post-movement" Chicano and Latino studies scholars have little patience with critics who mimic the nationalists of the 1960s. This doesn't mean that they reject all of their ideas; in fact, today's scholars and theorists embrace a number of assumptions underlying Chicano nationalism. But rather than wielding an essentialized conception of ethnic identity to serve as a kind of litmus test of one's "Mexicanness," they have fully complicated this model. The most discerning refuse to judge Mexican Americans on nationalistic assumptions, especially not those Mexican Americans of an earlier era, like Uncle Walker, who were actually raised under Jim Crow. Walker, in short, may get a well-deserved pass today.

Uncle Walker casts a long shadow over all Mexican Americans who inevitably confront their collective past. Successful and "assimilated," a man who carries within him a history that none of his two daughters' descendants will ever know and few privileged Mexican Americans today will ever see, his life captures the aggrieved struggle of first-generation Mexican Americans in the American wilderness. And despite all I have confessed about Walker, there is, of course, defiant heroism in his life, too, though expressed differently than by "movement" Chicanos. Even today, if the "brown plague" infects many of us because we share more in common with Uncle Walker than we care to admit, and if his life is somehow emblematic of a generation's struggle, then perhaps, rather than judging him in the manner of earlier critics, we should see in him a portrait of our buried past.

Part III

Race and Medicine

Race in medicine recapitulates race in America. Physicians require consultations from their colleagues in other fields of study—literature, anthropology, sociology, communication, Chicano studies, and the rest— as we evaluate how race is considered, and applied, in medicine. What is race? What isn't it? Race can be conflated with class, insurance status, education, and so on. "Diversity" itself is an ambiguous, treacherous, superficial idea. Decreasing inequalities in health for minorities, who are sicker in many of the studied areas—diabetes, heart disease, stage of cancer, and more—is a good financial idea. There is also a moral argument, too, to be made for providing appropriate care to people, independent of their race.

FIVE

The Patient in the Room

Enrique D. Rigsby

The only time I enjoyed a doctor's visit was when the doctor visited me. This phenomenon—for those born post-1970—was known as a "house call," when a doctor actually ventured from the office to treat a patient in the home.

I grew up in the San Francisco Bay area community of Vallejo, about thirty miles north of the city. In Vallejo, we had two "colored" doctors. Both were family friends, and for me and my brother, they were role models of what a child with my skin could become.

The house calls were made by Dr. Herman Williams—a tall, elegant, gentle man—who, if you asked my mother, had a Nat King Cole voice and a Billy Dee Williams smile. Our family loved Dr. Williams. He was sincere and soft-spoken, with seemingly impeccable clinical competence and the bedside manner of Mother Teresa. Each visit was an opportunity to remind us children that "Dr. Williams embodies the reason why you boys should do well in school—especially math and science," followed by a dose of our neighborhood's personal pledge: "And remember, once you get that education, no one can ever take it away from you."

Dr. Williams did not intimidate, nor did he pontificate to impress. We were valued human beings to him. I recall one house visit to treat my brother who was suffering with symptoms of the flu. Normally this would have been a rather routine appointment. However, it was in the mid-1960s, and the Hong Kong flu was epidemic. Dr. Williams not only treated my brother but also took time to discuss the disease, and the likelihood of the infection spreading to other family members. His job was rhetorical just as much as physical. Dr. Williams understood the importance of both. He would come out of his environment and enter our neighborhood, park in front of our house on Louisiana Street, walk into our home, venture into our bedroom, kneel down at our bedside, and talk gently about everything from the effects of the flu to the impact that consuming two dozen fruit pies in four hours can have on a digestive system. Dr. Williams discussed school, church, Little League, and what I wanted to be when I grew up. I am sure we were not his only patients, but the doctor never rushed, was never in a hurry.

I think my mother enjoyed his visits more than any of us. I must note that my mother was a happily married woman, and whenever Dr. Williams would come over, it was such a big deal that my father would take off work to be present. But I cannot help but share the following observations. I recall that when Dr. Williams arrived at our home, my mother was never in her mumu, nightgown, or robe. Her hair was never in curlers or covered with a do-rag. It wasn't the pearls and curls of June Cleaver, but close. Casual attire was replaced with Sunday dresses, red lipstick, and a few splashes of Jean Nate. She was never on the phone, nor did she entertain the inquiries of others who may have knocked at the front door. Viola Rigsby was front and center, present in the moment. The word "perky" might best describe my mother when Dr. Williams would arrive. Perky and very attentive!

Even Daddy stood up straight, because there was competition in the house. My father's appearance was more professional, his words more measured. It was quite obvious to me and my brother that medical royalty had descended upon our home, and we were expected to offer the appropriate responses—our very best behavior. When Dr. Williams came to visit, it was not the time for idle chatter, meaningless banter, or bathroom humor. We turned *The Three Stooges* off the television and spoke as if we were encyclopedia salesmen. Within our family, Herman Williams, MD, commanded the utmost respect.

In subsequent years, house calls became a distant memory. They vanished from the conscience of American culture right along with rotary-dial phones, the typewriter, and the transistor radio. The thought of a doctor making such a home visit today is unimaginable. Patient priority and convenience have given way to crowded schedules that produce more billable procedures, and illusions of self-importance that produce doctor-centered treatment.

As the years moved us from "naturals" and *Sanford and Son* to "Jeri-curls" and *The Cosby Show*, they also brought the declining health and eventual passing of my parents, and the valiant fight of a brave wife whose courage could not overcome the ravages of breast cancer. Losing Mom and Dad was overwhelming. Losing my wife, Trina, was devastating . . . horrifying. Trina—a registered nurse by vocation—battled for six years following the diagnosis. Within the first two weeks, Trina underwent a radical mastectomy, including the removal of twelve positive lymph nodes from tissue under her left arm. In an instant, Trina's identity changed from vibrant and healthy wife and mommy to a diagnosed and staged cancer patient whose remaining years would be spent in and out of oncology departments.

At age thirty-five, Trina was typically the youngest patient in the waiting room. Feeling more like audience members at a Tony Bennett concert, we managed to connect with our older comrades by swapping stories, sharing fears, and mostly reassuring each other that we would beat our common foe.

Being a cancer patient means your life is on hold. We quickly discovered that our time was no longer ours. The first sign of this was evident with our first trip to a specialist. The amount of time spent in a waiting room is tantamount to waiting at the Detroit airport for your delayed connection to Pasadena. We waited to see specialists, waited for radiation, waited for chemotherapy treatments, waited to talk with docs who always seemed to temper their optimism with lines like "Let's just wait and see how this works." I often wondered how the rhetoric and tone of doctors would change if more of them were cancer patients. I soon found myself resenting them, detesting their antiseptic and impersonal way of communicating.

From our experience, the dominant rhetorical features of a doctor's remarks were distant, clinical, uninviting, and most of all authoritative. For Trina and me, the language systematically and scientifically reduced us from humans to numbers—a case . . . dots on a probability chart that predicts and determines everything from how deep to cut, how much to poison, and how long to burn. Compassionate care gave way to medical jargon that included statistical probabilities and impersonal distance. Even Marcus Welby had a heart! Before long, we realized the game: The doctor must always be protected. And what better way to cover your speculations than to talk about the math and not the miraculous. Not exactly an environment of optimism, encouraging healing and hope. I began to realize that I was a long way from Louisiana Street, and these doctors, as nice as they tried to be, were no Herman Williams, MD.

I'd met Trina during my freshman year in college. She was the most beautiful woman I had ever met, and I wanted to be with her all the time. And if being with her meant I actually had to study . . . well, hello, Aristotle! Trina was preparing for a career in healthcare, and following school she found employment as a labor and delivery nurse at a local hospital. Following a career in television news, I returned to school for advanced degrees and eventual employment as a college professor of communication. At the time of Trina's diagnosis, therefore, we were well educated.

What's astonishing is that despite our educational backgrounds and life experiences, we never felt comfortable in the doctor's office. Practitioners were talking *at* us, rather than *to* us. Lost in a barrage of medical scripts, we seemed rather inconsequential to the "dialogue" occurring— as if we were two sponges there to absorb, and not to contribute. So we listened to diagnoses, treatment options, therapy schedules, and the like. My wife's medical background, her training and work as a registered nurse, even the fact that her brother was a board-certified orthopedic surgeon, offered little in the way of audience credibility to doctors whose discursive and non-discursive rhetorical choices suggested that any contribution from us would be meaningless. It reminded me of traveling to Texas, where my father had grown up, for family reunions each summer. I loved everything about those visits—except one little line that my aunts and uncles would repeat incessantly: *Children are to be seen and not heard.* This is *exactly* how Trina and I felt in the doctor's office.

In a strange way, I felt very much like the people I once reported on in my research as a doctoral student and civil rights scholar. My wife was diagnosed with cancer just months following the completion of my doctoral work in rhetorical theory with an emphasis in protest rhetoric. For the next two decades, I would study marginalized populations who responded to the exigencies of segregation in the hope of seeking redress from the established order. I could not help but wonder what it felt like to be marginalized. Sadly, it is a feeling I am all too familiar with. I also thought that if I was feeling as insecure and inadequate in the doctor's office—when I have a PhD, along with my wife, who was a nurse—what must the other patients who enter the office feel? What chance in the world do they have to contribute to the conversation about their healing and health? Perhaps the more critical question is: How do such rhetorical situations foster a context for disparities in the healthcare profession? Such a question, I would argue, calls for an examination of the role of rhetoric, in general, and the construction of power constituents versus subordinate roles, particularly within the context of the doctor's office.

Several years ago, while on the faculty at Texas A&M University, I was invited by a colleague to speak to her class, second-year medical students who were studying the communicative dimensions of health-care—presently among the most significant subspecialties of study in the communication discipline. I was not asked to speak because of my expertise in healthcare communication. Rather, I was asked to discuss how doctors might interact with terminally ill patients and their families. By now, Trina had passed away, and my colleague and friend thought this might be therapeutic for me and informative for the students.

I'll never know what impact I had on those students. My grief was profound and raw. I can report that after my presentation there were few dry eyes. I told students that for most of our six years in the healthcare system, we felt powerless and excluded from decisions that ranged from times for family vacations (always around chemo schedules) to what might be the best new therapy-related protocol to pursue. I shared with students that the roles are very clear: The doctor is the authoritative expert—challenge or question at your own expense. Also clear is that we are the patient in the room. And that patient is looking for two things: (1) clear answers to significant questions, and (2) the sound of anything that resembles hope.

In retrospect, now with over a decade to reflect, I think what would have helped Trina and me deal with the horrific destruction that cancer causes would have been more compassion. We never asked for medical practitioners to hide or mask the truth. But offer some compassion, some hope. We left most doctor visits depressed, discouraged, and deflated. A little bit of hope may not cure cancer, but it might encourage one to keep fighting.

I concluded my talk with the medical students by encouraging them to be extreme in their competence, and sincere in their compassion . . . as if it were their relative in the room.

In 1997, Barbara Sharf and Richard Street coauthored an article asserting that, traditionally, "social concerns of patients related to their health status are repeatedly marginalized and ignored by practitioners."[1] I wonder what the effect would be if those social dimensions were at least addressed. Is it plausible to suggest that patient satisfaction could be affected if doctors discussed social concerns? Could the enhancement of communicative dimensions such as language, participation, and inclusion increase the value of doctor-patient interaction? Could a physician's sensitivity to the patient's cultural values benefit patients and family members? These scholars call for a shift from the power imbalance of a biomedical model of interaction to one that gives a voice to patients.

I wonder how our experiences may have been different had practitioners used language that reflected inclusion and participation. They would speak about us and our lives and what they thought would be best for us. The only time we felt included or valued was when a particular nurse would linger following the "official" doctor visit to answer questions and share our concerns as best she could.

I don't recall ever having a conversation that included the quality of our lives. What I recall is the urgency to follow therapy protocols at all costs—usually rendering patients and family members powerless and frustrated.

Trina and I were used to a more personal, more informal mode of communication. This could be because we're African American. It could also be because of the type of people we are. We were a very outgoing, loving, and caring family unit. We loved people. I know that in my family, the dinner table was always the setting for a variety show! *Amateur Night at the Apollo* could not hold a candle to holidays with a house full of Rigsby relatives! A stringent, formalized, scripted, and linear mode of communication does not work for every patient. It certainly did not work for us. Realizing that people react and respond in different modes does not mean a physician has to reflect multiple personalities. However, it might suggest that the doctor could simply be a bit more humane in interactions.

A MORE HUMANE SYSTEM

Whatever happened to doctors such as Herman Williams? For that matter, where are the teachers, attorneys, and business moguls who place helping over profits, and compassion over compensation? The post–civil rights era produced significant change in America politically, legally, and socially as disenfranchised populations found a voice for redress through advocacy. Did a societal shift from needing an advocate one moment to screaming "Black Power" the next spark subtle changes in the way professionals are trained? When considering the broader societal landscape in America, our culture has produced a climate that seemingly ignores basic values such as helping and encouraging as normative behaviors among professional providers. It's all about being the "best" doctor, whether the kind portrayed at the local clinic or those who appear during an episode of *Grey's Anatomy*. Did the mandate for self-empowerment in the 1960s neuter professional training programs in ways that are less humane? Was assimilation into medical schools that produce "robots" trained to treat disease but not at the expense of showing too much compassion the price we paid? Trina and I needed a competent doctor *and* a compassionate friend. I can only wonder how our healthcare experience might have been different.

I am not naïve enough to believe that a greater display of compassion among physicians would have saved Trina's life. However, I would like to suggest that a slight shift from a biomedical communication model would have produced genuine encouragement during a time of great difficulty and tremendous uncertainty.

Moreover, assuming the role of patient as advocate would have encouraged our family to own a portion of the interactive process. As stakeholders with a voice, our contributions are meaningful and our opinions are valuable. The ability to have even a paucity of authority would generate a spirit of cooperation between patient and physician, creating the sense of a determined partnership that is ready to battle the enemy of disease.

Using language reflecting inclusion and participation would have resulted in a rich dialogue that would have been more reassuring, compassionate, and empathetic. Perhaps some doctors are insensitive to the realities of patients and family members who feel all alone, sense a loss of control, and are therefore extremely vulnerable and immensely overwhelmed.

It is incumbent upon medical schools to study the rhetorical dimensions of doctor-patient interactions—more specifically, a patient-centered model in which more than one stakeholder is identified, more than one person is honored, and more than one outcome is verbalized. The patient in the room is first and foremost a person . . . with logic and emotion and fears and hopes. Most of all, the patient in the room has *the* most vested interest in the outcome of all medical procedures. *Doctors, Px: Patients are to be seen . . . and heard!*

NOTE

1. Barbara F. Sharf and Richard L. Street Jr., "The Patient as Central Construct: Shifting the Emphasis," *Health Communication* 9, no. 1 (1997): 1–11.

SIX

Saying and Doing White Racism

Jennifer L. Pierce

Pueblo is a medium-sized town in southern Colorado about twenty miles east of the Rocky Mountains and one hundred miles south of Denver. When I was growing up, Coloradoans who came from Denver, or other more affluent areas to the north, called Pueblo "Pew town," as in "PU, it stinks," a reference to the smoke-belching steel mill that lies to the east side of I-25, the interstate that runs north and south through this town of 100,000 people. Until the economic recession of the mid-1970s, when most factory jobs in the steel industry were eliminated across the United States, Pueblo's local economy was dominated by the mill. The parents of most of my school friends worked at the mill, and, by the time I was in high school in the early 1970s, most of my male classmates assumed that they, too, would work there, unless they were lucky enough to get an athletic scholarship to attend college.

Pueblo's population was about 30 percent Mexican American, with a tiny percentage of African Americans and Native Americans. Everyone else was White—though no one I knew described him or herself that way. With last names like Oreskovich, Milisavljevich, Spinuzzi, Gagliardia, and Maguire, most claimed to be Polish, Italian, or Irish, which, as I learned later, were the very immigrant groups who had been recruited early in the twentieth century to work at the mill. Importantly, the Arkansas River, which runs through the center of Pueblo, was the dividing line between Mexico and the United States until 1848, when Mexico's northern territories (all or part of what is today Arizona, California, Colorado, Nevada, New Mexico, and Texas) were annexed to the United States under the Treaty of Guadalupe Hidalgo. If my family had lived in Pueblo before 1848, where I grew up on the south side of town, we would have been living in northern Mexico. My status as an American citizen, like that of many others, is an accident of historically contingent national boundaries.

Of course, this regional history was not taught in my local high school. What little I did know about American race relations came through my experiences living in Chicago, where my family had moved for three years so my dad could do a medical residency. We arrived in 1967 and moved back to Pueblo in 1969. During that time, Martin Luther King Jr. and Robert Kennedy were assassinated, and Chicago hosted the infamous 1968 Democratic Convention and one of the largest anti–Vietnam War protests in the country. My mother, who supported Eugene McCarthy, the antiwar candidate, thought Mayor Richard Daley and his "blue meanies" were idiots. She cried for days after King's assassination. Meanwhile, a number of public schools in Chicago lowered their flags to half-staff to honor King's memory, but the principal at our local grade school refused to do so. My mother, along with several other parents in our neighborhood, went to the grade school to complain.

"The god-damn-fuck-son-of-a-bitch better lower the flag to half-mast," she told my father before she stalked off to the meeting with some of our neighbors. Eventually, the principal complied. (I suspect he feared ending up on her "shit list," as did many who knew my mother well. Believe me, you did not want to end up on *that* list.) As it turned out, one neighbor was not pleased about the American flag flying at half-mast in front of Grand Avenue Elementary. Standing at our backdoor, Mrs. Smith hissed to my mother that King was a "commie Negro" and didn't deserve to be honored. While I stood in the background, my mother called Mrs. Smith a "bigot" and slammed the screen door in her fat, dough-colored face.

Later, over dinner of creamed chipped beef over toast, I asked my mother what the word "bigot" meant. "They're all a bunch of fucking idiots," she replied. My dad laughed at her remark, but then turned serious and explained that bigots were "bad people . . . bad White people who hated Black people." This didn't make much sense to my eight-year-old worldview, since I knew that White people like Bobby Kennedy got assassinated and antiwar protesters got beat up by the police during the Democratic Convention. "It's about race," my father explained. "Some people hate other people because they come from a different racial background."

"Hmm," I murmured, but did not say aloud, "that must be why Mom thinks Mrs. Smith is a fucking idiot."

What I took from all these experiences by the time we moved back to Pueblo was that American race relations were about Blacks and Whites. It wasn't until I was in high school that I thought much about the implications of racism for Mexican Americans. (One of those privileges of Whiteness: You don't have to think much about race because presumably it's not about you.) Racial slurs directed against Mexican Americans, such as "beaner," "greaser," and "spic," were common at my school, as were terms reserved for White ethnics, such as "Polack." Another series of ethnic jokes that circulated with great frequency were called "Bojon jokes" (pronounced bō-jŏn). Like many other ethnic and racial jokes, the punch line establishes the stupidity of the "Bojon" by showing that he does not understand some piece of conventional wisdom. Not until graduate school did I discover that the term "Bojon" is actually an abbreviation for "born on journey," a reference to all kinds of racially and ethnically "suspect migrants"—people from Southern and Eastern Europe along with those from Mexico and Asia who were born in transit to the United States. At the time, I knew these were all pejorative terms, and I am sure they had always been in use, but their prevalence and ugly meaning didn't sink in until they implicated someone I knew.

In grade school, one of my friends (and as a shy, bookwormish twelve-year-old, I didn't have many friends) was a girl named Kathy Martinez. Whenever I went over to her house, Kathy's mother sent me home with homemade beef flautas left over from lunch and wrapped in tinfoil for my family. When Kathy came to our house, my mother, who hated to cook, but was not to be outdone in working-class norms of reciprocity, sent Kathy home with a warm, brown paper bag full of homemade chocolate chip cookies. By the end of sixth grade, Kathy and I ended up going to different middle schools, and by high school, where several different middle school populations merged, we never found ourselves in the same classroom, though I sometimes saw her in the hallways with her new group of friends and we casually waved hello to one another.

Her new set of friends, mostly Mexican American, were all enrolled in what were then termed "vocational track classes." Remember typing, bookkeeping, and machine shop? Between classes, they hung out and sometimes smoked in the school's quadrangle outside. A group of stoners, my younger brother among them, also hung out on the quad. I, too, had a new set of friends. Some were on the track team, and after school each spring we spent hours running laps, doing jumping jacks and push-ups, and practicing for our meets. (The coach had determined that my long, gangly legs were best suited for the 440 and the long jump.) The rest of my friends—the brainy ones—were on the editorial board of the school newspaper. Although they weren't all White, particularly on the track team, most were Italian, Irish, or Polish American. In this way, the racial and ethnic sorting through guidance counselor "suggestions" for different educational tracks and friendship patterns had begun to emerge.

At some point in my freshman year, my mother learned that Kathy's father had been ill and could no longer work at the mill. By the early 1970s, the mill had already eliminated about one-third of its positions through downsizing. The parents of some of my friends were already unemployed and looking for work. So it was unlikely that there would be a job at the mill when he got better—if indeed his health improved. My mother prepared a Hamburger Helper casserole and put it in a large Tupperware container, and then we drove over to Kathy's house.

When we arrived, Kathy's mother ushered us into the kitchen, and when she opened their refrigerator, I saw that it was already filled with other Tupperware containers and a variety of mystery shapes wrapped in tinfoil. Meanwhile, Mark Spinuzzi, one of the star basketball players from our high school team—and a senior, no less—was out back mowing their lawn; a number of other adults from the neighborhood were talking out on the back stoop. As my mother spoke in hushed tones to Mrs. Martinez, she, in turn, told me that Kathy was in her room.

I quickly exited the world of adult conversation and went into Kathy's bedroom, the very room where we had listened to 45s on her record player in sixth grade and sang along to the Monkeys: "*Hey, hey, we're the Monkeys, people say we monkey around, but we're too busy singing, to let anybody get us down.*" Kathy was sitting in front of a mirror attached to a vanity table, brushing her long, dark brown hair. She smiled sadly when she saw me. I had no idea what to say. Her father was in the hospital, and the doctors had not yet confirmed what we all found out later: he had lung cancer, a cancer that may have been caused by the carcinogenic fumes he breathed every day at the mill for twenty years. I stood at her doorway, hesitantly smiling and waiting.

Kathy finally said, "So, did you see that Mark Spinuzzi is in the backyard mowing the lawn?"

I nodded, thinking how lucky she was to have one of the most popular and handsome seniors in her backyard. Seniors rarely bothered to talk to freshmen like me. "I didn't know you knew him."

"His family lives down the block. Did you know he and his dad call us beaners?"

"What?"

"Yeah, they call us beaners, and now he's out back mowing the lawn. His mom even brought over a pan of homemade ravioli."

"What an asshole!"

"Yeah, he's an asshole all right. I told my mom he has to pull all the dandelions, too."

I laughed. The idea that one of the most popular boys in the senior class had to mow the Martinezes' lawn and pull weeds seemed a just punishment.

Finally, I said, "Sorry about your dad."

"Thanks."

After an awkward silence, Kathy said, "So, what did your mom bring over?"

"Hamburger Helper casserole."

"What! No chocolate chip cookies?"

I laughed and said, "Actually, your mom's flautas were always the best."

Kathy smiled and said, "Yeah, they were always in that Greatest Mom sweepstakes. Whose mom can provide the best homemade food for the other family?"

From the kitchen, I heard my mother calling, "Jenny, time to go."

"Well," I said, "I'll see you around."

"Yeah," Kathy said. "Maybe." Then she quickly added, "Hey, tell your mom thanks. But next time, I want chocolate chip cookies."

That night at home for dinner we ate the other Tupperware container of Hamburger Helper along with canned green beans and an iceberg lettuce salad covered with bottled French dressing, followed by strawberry Jell-O topped with Cool Whip for dessert. My mom told my dad about visiting Mrs. Martinez. As I listened to her talk about all the neighbors who had pitched in to help, I finally interjected, "But they're not really so great. Mark and his dad call the Martinezes beaners."

"What!" my mom exclaimed.

"Hmm," my dad said.

"Yeah, and Kathy said that she's going to make him pull weeds, too. He and his dad are assholes."

"Language," my mom said. My mother maintained a very strict double standard. She could swear like a sailor, as my dad often pointed out, but my brother and I were not supposed to use *that* kind of language.

"Jennifer," my father began.

Uh oh, I thought. Any discussion with my father that began with "Jennifer" meant that I was about to receive a lecture on self-improvement.

"Although I don't approve of the language that Mr. Spinuzzi and his son used, I think you need to think about the things their family did for Mrs. Martinez."

I stared at the green beans growing cold on my plate.

"It's not just about what people say; it's also about what they do."

"But they said shitty things."

"Language!" my mom said.

My dad said, "Yes, they did. But they also brought food over to the house and helped with some of the chores that Mrs. Martinez doesn't have time to do now that her husband is in the hospital."

"That doesn't make it OK."

"No, it doesn't make it OK. But sometimes actions speak louder than words."

"Mowing the grass is better than hurting Kathy's feelings?"

"I know what they said hurt Kathy's feelings. But, in the meantime, the lawn got mowed, the weeds get pulled, and Mrs. Martinez has one less thing to worry about."

I pondered this, but it still didn't seem right.

A number of academic works explain the resurgence of the Republican Right in the 1980s by pointing the finger at disgruntled, White working-class men. As the argument goes, in books such as Thomas Frank's *What's the Matter with Kansas*, White working-class men were dissatisfied with the Democrats' lack of attention to their lives after the economic recession in the 1970s. They turned to Republicans in droves in the 1980s to support candidates whom they imagined appealed to their interests on racially divisive issues such as crime, welfare, and affirmative action. But what these academic studies seldom consider is the point my father made many years ago. On the one hand, White working-class Americans are more likely than their middle-class counterparts to provide unedited accounts of racism. At the same time, working-class norms of mutual aid and reciprocity sometimes contradict these espoused racist comments and views. Studies of White working-class racism rarely explore the meanings or consequences of these kinds of contradictions.

I started graduate school in the Department of Sociology at the University of California, Berkeley, in 1981. In my second year, I landed a job as a teaching assistant for Professor Harry Edwards, who taught an enormous undergraduate course on "The Sociology of Sport" in an auditorium seating five hundred students. Edwards has done pioneering research about how professional sports such as football and basketball reproduce racial inequality in the United States. This was the central theme of his academic course. His interest in race and sport drew from his own experiences as a Black student athlete, and he, along with Tommie Smith and John Carlos, were the political organizers for the Olympic Project for Human Rights that led to Smith and Carlos's infamous Black Power salute on the winners' podium at the 1968 Olympics. I should also mention that, in addition to being African American, Professor Edwards was about six feet, eight inches tall. He shaved his head and typically sported a black turtleneck sweater along with a black leather jacket and dark slacks. He was incredibly smart and, in terms of style, Black Panther cool—a style point that Berkeley undergraduates were unlikely to miss.

I suspect that many undergraduates thought the course would be an "easy A." After all, what could be so hard about a class on sports? Many were flummoxed by their low grades after the first midterm. Students whose papers I had been assigned to read came to complain to me about their grades in the box-sized office I shared with another teaching assistant.

"But I'm planning to go to law school," one White fraternity boy in navy blue and white striped Adidas flip-flops, shorts, and a T-shirt told me. "I have to get an 'A' in this course."

"This was a 'B–' exam," I replied. "The question you should be asking is how you can do better on your next essay exam."

He frowned at me, got up from his chair, and flip-flopped out the door.

About a week after the midterm, the three other teaching assistants and I arrived in the auditorium and took our seats near the back. Sitting in the back gave us an opportunity to "shush" those students who rudely conversed with one another during class. As Edwards began speaking, we noticed that a few students trickling in late came in and sat in the first row near the podium. Two of them wore dark blue T-shirts, jeans, and gorilla masks.

"What the fuck are they doing?" I asked Mike, the White TA sitting next to me, although I knew that at the height of college campus "culture wars," when other faculty of color, feminists, and Marxists were under attack by conservative students and intellectuals, students wearing gorilla masks to an African American professor's class obviously meant they intended to cause trouble.

"I don't know," he said, "but this is a problem."

Mike and I stood up and began moving our way through the legs of a long row of undergraduates, and then began to hurry down the stairs toward the front of the vast lecture hall. Meanwhile, a number of undergraduates began to laugh. Professor Edwards, never one to be at a loss for words, interrupted the opening of his lecture, glared sternly at the students, and said, "And what are you doing here today?" As Mike and I moved toward the front row hoping to persuade the two gorilla-masked bandits to leave, they stood up and scurried toward one of the auditorium exits.

"Some people just don't know what to do with themselves," Edwards said. The lecture hall rocked with laughter. Once it died down, he proceeded with the rest of his lecture.

In a discussion later in the day over a pitcher of cheap beer in a local Berkeley dive filled with sticky tables and a haze of cigarette smoke, the two other TAs proffered their critical analyses of these two students' theatrics. Neil explained that in the early twentieth century, particularly among some prominent anthropologists, as well as in the eugenics movement in the United States, African Americans were portrayed as closer to their simian evolutionary cousins than Caucasians, a racist assumption suggesting that they were less evolved as a racial group than other groups. Clearly, argued Tom, another TA, the gorilla-masked students had seized upon this simian metaphor in an effort to disrupt the class of an influential Black professor.

Though I did not disagree with his comments, I had to stifle a growing feeling of unease. Neil and the other TA had stayed lazily in their chairs to watch the show during the lecture while Mike and I had moved to the front of the room to do something—though I can't say we had an effective plan in mind. In addition, the other TAs all mysteriously disappeared after class. (Typically, we all checked in with the professor after class.) On this particular day, Mike and I were the only ones who remained to talk with Professor Edwards. When we spoke to him, we learned that he was grimly amused by the students' antics, but he explained it away by saying he had experienced "much worse." Knowing a bit of his political career, I imagined this was true, but to my way of thinking, that didn't make what the students did OK. Meanwhile, now in the safety of another locale far from this contentious event, these TAs, two young White men, both from privileged backgrounds, pontificated in a self-satisfied way about their interpretation of what had happened.

"So, how did Professor Edwards feel about this?" asked Maria, a Chicana graduate student who had joined us to hear about the latest in the "culture wars" on campus.

While the other TAs shifted around uncomfortably in their seats, Mike explained that Professor Edwards hadn't seemed that upset and had told us this wasn't a big deal compared to other experiences in his life. I added that it was disturbing, nonetheless, even if Edwards didn't make a big deal about it "to me and Mike." As I emphasized these last four words, I looked over at the disappearing TAs.

Maria turned to the other two men and asked, "So, what did he say to you?"

"Hey," Neil said. "I wasn't there. We all have other stuff to do. Besides, it's Harry's class and he's a big guy. He can take care of himself."

Maria stared at him and said, "So, you thought it was OK to leave after an auditorium filled with students laughed in his face?"

"Hey, you're getting this all wrong," Tom, the other TA, said. "Not everyone laughed."

"Besides," said Marsha, another White student who had joined the group, an Ivy League graduate who claimed to have been a Maoist as an undergraduate, "when Edwards got denied for tenure, everyone knows he called in President [Jimmy] Carter to support him. It's not like he's a sociological giant or anything."

I didn't see the relevance of Marsha's comment to Maria's question, but thought that she, Neil, and Tom were behaving like assholes.

"So, you all sit here drinking beer and offering your smug intellectual critique of what happened today, but none of you said anything at the time?" Maria asked, looking around the table.

Neil closely examined the bottom of his plastic beer stein. Mike and Tom gazed silently across the room. I shrugged, as if to say, "What else could we do?"

She glared at all of us, grabbed her book bag, and stalked out of the bar.

"What's her problem?" Neil asked.

Susan, another White graduate student who had joined us in the bar, said, "Did you know she changed her name from Jane to Maria?"

"Yeah, right, so she'd sound more ethnic," Marsha added, grinning. She and Susan laughed together as if sharing a private joke.

"Who cares what her name is?" Tom said. "I, for one, think she's really hot."

Disgusted by their remarks, I muttered the comment "asshole" in Tom's direction, stood up, pulled a few dollars out of my pocket, threw them on the table, and followed Maria's retreating back out of the bar.

"Hey, wait up," I said, when I got outside and saw her rushing along Telegraph Avenue. She turned around and flashed me a dirty look.

"Maria," I said. "They're all a bunch of assholes."

She turned around and said, "And you're not?"

Puzzled and hurt, and wondering how I had suddenly become one of the "bad guys," I could only stand open-mouthed and listen as she added, "I didn't hear you say anything to support me when I challenged them."

"But I don't agree with them," I said. "They are all fucking idiots."

"But you didn't say anything," she said. "If you don't stand up to people like that, you're just reinforcing the status quo."

A few years later, I began my dissertation research focusing on the workplace lives of women and men who worked as paralegals and lawyers in the San Francisco Bay area. At the time, I was still a novice researcher and harbored many doubts about my academic abilities. Though I had com-

pleted my required coursework and exams, I was among the few graduate students whose parents, though upwardly mobile, hailed from working-class backgrounds. Doing fieldwork in a predominantly White and
upper-middle-class milieu provoked my anxieties about saying the "right
thing."

On my first day in the field, I spent two and a half hours in the human
resources office filling out required paperwork, getting my picture taken
for my photo identification badge, and reading the company's literature
on affirmative action. As part of my induction, the tall brunette personnel
director, dressed in a severe navy blue skirt suit with matching low-
heeled pumps, ushered me into an empty office and turned on the VCR
for my "required" viewing of a twenty-minute video on the company's
affirmative action program. Her lined white face and brown eyes were
tightly pinched in a dark frown. After she left, I sat in the semi-darkened
room watching the opening scene: a factory floor filled with the smiling
faces of African American men and women operating heavy machinery
as a White man in a wheelchair answered phones. In the background, a
soft, cheerful, female voice said, "At ____ Corporation, we value diversity
and excellence." The upbeat video continued by promoting the "great
success" of the company's affirmative action program by showing foot-
age of more smiling faces of White women, Latinos, Asian Americans,
and African Americans in a variety of clerical and factory jobs.

The narrator proceeded to describe the beginning of the company's
affirmative action program fifteen years earlier. In her upbeat description
of the company's program, she failed to mention what I would later learn
from others: A federal court had ordered the corporation to create an
affirmative action program in response to a lawsuit filed against the company in the early 1970s for race *and* sex discrimination. The court's ruling
was based on a documented pattern of differential treatment in hiring
and promotion. When the video concluded, I walked back into the personnel director's office to fill out the remaining paperwork. The stat-
uesque, frowning brunette was no longer there, but her blonde assistant,
whose pixie-sized nose was decorated with a sprinkle of freckles, looked
up with a broad smile and asked if I had any questions. Puzzled by some
of what I had learned in the video, I asked, "Isn't it true that courts don't
mandate programs unless there's been a finding of 'egregious discrimination'?" I was surprised when this unknown, young White woman began

a verbal tirade against the corporation's affirmative action plan. She blamed it for mandating the hiring of "lots of unqualified minorities."[1]

Neglecting my avowed research commitment to being a "neutral" observer, I angrily replied that her comment was a racist one, adding that it also seemed to violate the very message of the video I had been viewing. Red-faced, she in turn replied, after glancing at my resume, "Oh, you went to Berkeley, didn't you?"

Over the following months, I learned that this one White woman's comment was only one piece of a broader hostile climate directed against BC's affirmative action program. My field notes from the time are filled with negative comments about the alleged effects of the program. In the legal department where I did my fieldwork, some of the White male lawyers complained about "those unqualified clerks in the file room" who, as I observed, just happened to be Black and Latino. In fact, the adjective "unqualified" popped up time and time again in casual conversations. Job candidates with unremarkable previous job histories were "unqualified" when they were people of color, but could use a "boost up" if they were White men. By this time, I had learned to keep my mouth shut during these conversations and dutifully recorded them in my field notes. Unlike the personnel assistant, however, these upper-middle-class White men did not attach the term "unqualified" to the word "minority." Instead, "unqualified" stood alone as a coded and pejorative signifier for people of color.

The White male attorneys' decision, as well as that of the personnel assistant, to share their opinion with me about affirmative action suggests that they all assumed we would share a similar viewpoint on this public policy. Since I was brand new to the workplace, the only basis for this assumption appeared to lie in our shared racial identities. Because I was White, they assumed I would share their point of view on affirmative action. When I did not, in the case of the personnel assistant, she looked for another reason to explain—and dismiss—my opinion.

Methodological work in sociology, at that time, suggested that "insiders" (people who shared the same gender or racial and ethnic background as their research subjects) had a number of advantages in doing their research. In sharing a similar background, they would presumably be more attuned to the worldviews and experiences of those they studied and, hence, produce more accurate research. Others argued that insiders carried with them an implicit bias in studying people like themselves.

These scholars argued that White scholars, unlike Black academics, for example, studying African Americans were more capable of meeting the academic norms of "objectivity" and "neutrality."

While the simplistic dichotomy of the "insider-outsider" debate has been challenged in recent years, what is important to consider about the historical moment in which this academic discussion took place is that many White sociologists studied White people, but *their* "objectivity" was seldom questioned. In fact, until the early 1990s, whiteness as a social category received little attention in academic research. Most of the scholarly work on race in the United States presumed that race was a "marked" social category signifying people of color. Pioneering studies such as historian David Roediger's *The Wages of Whiteness* and sociologist Ruth Frankenburg's *White Women, Race Matters: The Social Construction of Whiteness* challenged this assumption by asking researchers to conceptualize whiteness as a racial category that confers considerable advantages in one's life chances. The central thrust of scholarship in critical whiteness studies is to render this previously unmarked racial category *visible* as a central organizing principle in social and cultural relations of racial inequality.

Many years later, as a tenured professor, I began conducting research for a book on the backlash against affirmative action in California in the 1990s. I reinterviewed the male and female lawyers I had first spoken to in the late 1980s. By 1999, when I talked with them again, Proposition 209, the so-called civil rights initiative banning the consideration of race and gender in education, employment, and contracting, had passed in California. In this historical context, a professional workplace with a federally mandated affirmative action program seemed a timely window into White professionals' understanding of racial inequality, as well as a means of making whiteness visible.

Though the majority of attorneys were White in this legal department of 150 lawyers, there were three lawyers of color. Randall Kingsley, one of the African American attorneys I interviewed, described the behavior of the White male lawyers he worked with as "racing for innocence." For him, this phrase described liberal, professional, upper-middle-class, White men who espoused "color blindness," but in their daily workplace practices either failed to mentor or excluded people of color in informal professional socializing.[2]

As I did more interviews, I found that Kingsley's phrase aptly described a more general pattern of color-blind language and racially exclusionary practices among this group of professional White elites. These White men, who were uncomfortable discussing race, were also quick to disavow their accountability for racism, while at the same time they did little to support or include people of color in their workplace.

This distinction between what White people say and what they do has long been at the back of my mind since my father and I had our discussion about the working-class families in our neighborhood who supported the Martinez family. While I was critical at the time of what I understood to be hypocritical behavior by some, my father reminded me to think about what people did and what they said and what mattered most for neighbors in times of crisis. Many academic studies on White racism tend to focus their blame on White working-class Americans. They have become the evil villains in a story about the backlash against affirmative action and the resurgence of the Republican Right in the 1980s and beyond.

What these same studies fail to consider is the fact that White upper-middle-class men and women are far more "polite" or "careful" about how they discuss racial issues in our post–civil rights era of "color blindness." They may *say* that they believe individuals should be judged by their talents and accomplishments, and not by the color of their skin, but what do they actually *do*? Research shows that most White, middle-class Americans choose to live in predominantly White neighborhoods, marry spouses of their own racial and ethnic background, oppose affirmative action, and, if given the opportunity, hire employees like themselves rather than African Americans or Latinos. These facts were true of almost all the White lawyers I interviewed.

More significantly, these professional elites wield greater power than their working-class counterparts in determining who will be hired, retained, and promoted in workplaces. And, as attorneys, they have far more influence in the United States than many other workers: They participate in lobbying efforts to buttress the interests of corporations; as members of Congress, they create social policies that have reduced federal subsidies to poor people; and as judges, they have interpreted and decided laws that restrict the use of the term "class" in antidiscrimination suits (for example, the 2011 *Wal-Mart* Supreme Court decision). Collectively, the lawyers I studied, as well as the legal profession itself, more broadly maintain and reproduce whiteness as a structure of power and privilege.

Of course, one might argue that White working-class folks are also involved in reproducing the racial status quo, and that I have presented an overly romanticized view of neighborly mutual aid. After all, many of these White men who were previously solid Democrats crossed over in the 1980s to vote for Republican candidates who promised to be "tough on crime" (or, as Republican political ads suggested, to put "criminal" people of color in jail), to eliminate welfare for "undeserving" women of color, and to abolish "unfair racial preferences" in hiring and promotion. My intent is not to deny the racism either in the framing of these political issues or in how many working-class Americans responded to them. Rather, my interest lies in painting a more complicated portrait of White racism that illuminates the messiness of lived realities that are often flattened out or lost in sociological surveys of racial attitudes or in historical research relying on voting patterns.

What my personal observations suggest is that what White people say and what they do takes on distinct forms among different socioeconomic groups with divergent consequences. As my father said long ago, in spite of the ugly things the Spinuzzi men said about the Martinez family, Mrs. Martinez got her lawn mowed and her neighbors brought over food and comfort; although her husband later died, many working-class neighbors from various racial and ethnic backgrounds continued to support her family in the ways that their own limited circumstances made possible: a ride to the hospital, a bag of groceries, a pan of ravioli, a Tupperware container of Hamburger Helper.

The White lawyers I interviewed, on the other hand, rarely used racial slurs, professed their belief in equal opportunity, but did little to mentor or support attorneys of color. Despite their disavowals of racism, they did *nothing* to create a more inclusive workplace. In fact, by doing nothing, wittingly or not, they participated in the backlash against affirmative action. My White, self-described liberal-to-radical colleagues in graduate school participated in a similar contradictory dynamic: They proffered critiques of racism, but did little to challenge the status quo, and, as Maria aptly observed, my silence reproduced the same problem.

Racism is certainly not unique to White middle-class or upper-middle-class Americans. Many White working-class Americans are involved in efforts to marginalize people of color, and some people of color are quick to undermine other minoritized racial groups when it is advanta-geous to do so. My point is slightly different: Which group of people has the most power to make a difference? Mowing a lawn for a family or bringing them food and comfort is kind and generous during a time of crisis, but these activities didn't help Mrs. Martinez find a good job with health insurance after her husband died of lung cancer. With the steel mill operating at one-third of its former capacity by the late 1970s, none of the working-class adults I knew were in a position to offer her a job. Middle-class White folks who could didn't bother.

NOTES

1. Jennifer L. Pierce, *Gender Trials: Emotional Lives in Contemporary Law Firms* (Berkeley and Los Angeles: University of California Press, 1995), 201.

2. For a full discussion of this one attorney's experiences, see Jennifer L. Pierce, *Racing for Innocence: Whiteness, Gender, and the Backlash against Affirmative Action* (Stanford, CA: Stanford University Press, 2012), 64–83.

SEVEN

Fred Sanford's People Are from St. Louis

Richard Garcia

I tell people that I'm Mexican. I generally don't start things this way, however. I usually say enough words, give enough clues, that this classification of mine, if we must, becomes clear within the context of my narrative. Or else, if in the natural progression of a conversation with someone who doesn't know—whether they're interested isn't quite the question for me—I find that mentioning I'm Mexican is germane, then I do. To keep the narrative going. But not as its denouement. More as a datum as we discuss something important.

And then there's how I look. I wrote that sentence using the passive verb tense, as it's not something anyone can really actively construct. I mean beyond dress and appearances. Style and behavior. Stereotype, then, of what's expected. I look Mexican. All right. Or else Native American, which gets to be the same thing, depending upon where we draw lines inside of American history.

I try not to push this too far, since I've never been to Mexico, don't speak Spanish, am not Catholic, and such. Thus, I meet none of the qualifications for being Mexican.

Other than being Mexican, that is.

I was born in Stockton, California, where my mother was born, and where her mother, too, was born. Things become vague beyond this part of my family history. They also become Mexico. Nevertheless, I only speak English.

And I believe in nothing.

Discussions about race can be tiresome, or, rarely, if they are good ones, fiery. I enjoy them in the right hands. Essays about race, however, are typically just tiresome. (I'll do what I can, here, to keep people around.)

I recall a sign on a water tower from about the eighth grade: "Stockton, Someplace Special." I didn't know if it was true. Nor would its truth have mattered, since Stockton was all I had in mind. The world, entirely, for me. I think there's a hockey league sign-up now. Maybe it's a Single A baseball team advertisement for the Stockton Ports. (I fondly remember them as the Mudville Ports from childhood.) Either way, the "Stockton, Someplace Special" sign is painted over. Brighter. What replaces the content of the nostalgic sign in my mind, at least, is a 2011 Forbes.com report claiming that Stockton is the most miserable city in America for the second time in three years. (While these rankings aren't official, they do place my city into context.) And since I come from the worst side of this certifiably miserable city, the math becomes even more oppressive.

I live in a pleasant city now, without crime. All right.

But *my* city is a Mexican and Black 1970s government duplex painted beige with brown trim. We moved to Fourth Street, across from Kenji Kobayashi, a Japanese guy, the summer before the sixth grade. I never considered being Mexican as its own entity during childhood. Kenji and I played doubles tennis with two kids who lived on Fifth Street. I had the best serve. Boy Cabangbang, a Filipino, had the best backhand. The three of us, with Timmy Ting, Boy's Chinese neighbor, created teams that made sense. Whether my serve was precise mattered most. It must have been in a sociology class as a Berkeley undergrad when I recognized that I'd played tennis with three Asian Americans. What I understood about race then, and now, for that matter, was that if we were to have any chance at all, I had better serve to Boy's forehand.

I believe I was still at Berkeley when I first heard the term "Hispanic." My "Hispanic" classmates and I quickly dismissed this sort of thing. And Berkeley professors taught us better. But the term was taking hold across the country, against my silent protest, I was to find.

During medical school in Chicago, on the last day of my psychiatry rotation, our professor offered to take three of us to lunch. Free food is priceless to medical students. (It turns out this is also true for residents in training and practicing doctors.) The psychiatry professor asked what we'd like to eat.

Anything would do.

The professor asked, "How about Cuban food?"

We all agreed. We walked to the nearby Cuban restaurant in downtown Chicago. I whispered to one of my psych classmates in the biting cold, "What do Cubans eat?"

The professor overheard me. "You don't know? But you're Hispanic! They eat black beans!"

I worried as we got closer to the Cuban restaurant, and recalled the only time I'd ever known black beans was when my California mother burned the pintos.

Why should I know about the habits of a Cuban who grew up in Puerto Rico and lives in Los Angeles? We are connected only by a linguistic conquest in antiquity. Yet, today, we live inside the Venn diagram of an American history class. I admit, although I don't speak Spanish, I do recognize our collective. In English.

"Latino" didn't quite take, either. It is a virtual vestige from antiquity's language culminating in the present children of conquistadors who only speak English. And for other reasons, classifying me as Latino misses the mark on my forehead.

Antiquity, perfectly formed, it seems, is what we can count on in the end.

My interest in "race," let's call it, peaked during my late undergraduate years. I later remained supplied by PBS documentaries, chatter with friends, occasional national news events, California ballots to expel Mexicans, and my own interaction with Mexicans from Mexico and from California, where our congruence remained in question.

In short, I'd moved on, I suppose.

My wife, who is Black, and I waited for our first baby. I understand this is an uncommon sociological location in America. Nevertheless, of all the things we'd imagined, much like all other parents, we wanted a full-term, healthy baby. This is what we got. Although we'd never really talked about the baby's would-be color, we both quietly and separately assumed the obvious: We'd have a brown baby—some unspoken color between mine and my wife's. She delivered our daughter: reddish hair, blue-gray eyes, and white skin. (Ultimately, against all medical judgment as a pediatrician, I ordered a blood test to see if she was anemic. She was not. White was her color, medically speaking.) Two months later, my wife walked the baby into her pediatrician's office where another mother looked down at them both and said, "Don't worry, she'll darken up."

We don't worry. We don't talk about color in our house. Except as grace notes in substantive conversations. And for fun. My wife gave a picture of our baby to her aunt, who placed it on top of the TV. When my wife's uncle walked downstairs, he said, "Who is this Irish baby you have on top of the TV?" Even now, fourteen years later, when he sees our daughter at a family party, my wife's uncle says to our daughter, "Top of the morning to you!"

We laugh.

Our daughter doesn't get it.

Our son looks approximately like her, but with brown eyes.

Our third, and final, baby came out brown. She looks like the other two. (My friend, a Harvard neonatologist who wondered how we kept creating these white babies, said about the brown baby's picture I sent him, "I knew you could do it!")

Our children are simple scientific possibilities inside of American history.

I failed when I detailed to my friend, an electrical engineer from India and Stanford, that I don't speak Spanish; I don't know what Cubans eat; I don't know what it means to leave my country; I'm not Catholic; I hold no special place in my heart for the Queen of Spain; I read James Baldwin's essays; my children don't quite know they're Black, and they don't quite know they're Mexican because the evidence presented to their young minds controverts these fictions—fictions they will learn soon enough. Our daughter, a toddler who knows her colors, says I'm brown. In fact, she is correct. We will further correct her as she gets older. Ordinary living, too, will correct our unsuspecting children.

My own concept of race has its origins in my high school—Filipino, Mexican, Japanese, Black, Chinese, White, for the most part—though I'd forgotten about my Indian friend until our recent high school reunion, where I recognized him as Indian now that I've known Indians in medicine, although before I had only ever known him as Kanwal. His British accent was more obvious to me at our reunion as adults, having seen *Bend It Like Beckham* and such by now. I went back and found that my childhood neighborhood is different. The old one remains in my mind, however. What is the social context of race for my children? That we improved their class makes all the difference, I'm told.

Then "race" cannot exist in colloquial terms. But we talk about race, and it does exist as a metaphysical conundrum, a brainteaser, a non sequitur.

It turns out that one drop does not maketh the Negro. Race, Black fathers, White mothers, melanin, genetic lineage, conquistadors, Thomas Jefferson, and other anthropological and overt historical tricks are on hand in our common language about race in America. One of my colleagues, as we discussed health disparities between the races in America, said about my white-appearing Black children, "We may have to leave them out of this discussion. But America knows who the rest of us are. They knew it when they threw us off the front of the bus."

Naturally, there are no White people in Europe. Only French, Italian, Irish, German, Dutch, and the like. And there are no Black people in Africa—only Nigerians, Kenyans, and Egyptians, who seem to have no interest in my wife's family's journey from Mississippi to Chicago to Los Angeles. I never paid much attention to this until my medical school classmate went to Lagos, Nigeria, for a surgery elective during our senior year in medical school. A Nigerian surgeon jokingly (I think) said to him, "Don't come over here looking for your roots. You'd better go to Mississippi for that."

I reminded my friend of that episode of *Sanford and Son* when Lamont wore a dashiki as he searched for his African roots. Fred Sanford declined the search, and noted that his people are from St. Louis.

I am a Mexican, by all accounts. But to be Mexican from Stockton in modern America is to exist in a state of alterity, if at all. In terms that are not my own, no matter my protest. Identity, which always seemed so active to me, ignites an interior monologue when we wake from sleep. Step outside. Or remain inside, invisible in any case. Passive, then.

A chapter on race in a medical book might contain attempts at genetic definitions, allele changes, chimpanzee versus people comparisons, percentages of genetic similarity above 99 percent, with all the other human variance to be determined by the remaining fictional 1 percent, or less. Such a chapter could examine Puerto Rican genes and compare and contrast them with those of Mexican people or Black people or Spanish people, as if the author was about to discover something circa 1600 to explain American social variance as was seen by the naked eye then, and by DNA sequencing techniques now.

But this is not the point.

A Black woman with breast cancer is likely to have a more aggressive cell type as compared with a White woman. This fact is uncontroverted. (Let's leave aside, for now, that the Black woman is likely to have lived closer to toxins and to have received a late diagnosis, is less likely to have had screening mammograms to intercept this late diagnosis, and is statistically less able to have health insurance that would mitigate the cost to her and her family, and to us all.) The scientific fact that cancerous cell types from the two *groups* of women biologically behave differently is uninteresting when it comes to her *particular* cell type and her *particular, tangible* treatment. And that the care she can expect to receive, independent of the cell's aggressive nature, isn't the best possible care on earth, even if it is the most expensive.

Certainly, this is the line of discussion that can be expected in such a chapter. But when talking about race here, of all places, I'm necessarily drawn back home as I consider which possibilities exist, and which are out of reach.

I don't hope that people would read my chapter and think, *Gee, you know, the guy's right. Let's not label people anymore.* Or worse — *So, race doesn't exist?* Or even — *So, it exists. Now what?*

For me, I'll do my best to rear my children to live with my natural-born skepticism. Alas, the world will view them. Our eldest daughter is currently consumed with Greek mythology, Irish history, Chinese history, and the American Revolution. When she's older, I suspect she'll follow my urgings to review Frederick Douglass's narrative, to study Paul Robeson, to follow the old leftist edict — "Don't Fight Down" — and to read Baldwin to the point of being able to quote long passages at will. She and I met Richard Rodriguez for dinner in New York two weeks ago. She read his first book. She'll read more later. He signed his new book, *Darling: A Spiritual Autobiography*, for her: "Take the Future!" Our son is already indifferent, which I admire. And our brown youngest plans to major in coloring!

Their present childhoods invite me to consider my own childhood. As children, my cousins and I were nothing alike. The eldest was seven or eight years older than me. When I was eight, and he was fifteen or sixteen, "growing up together" wasn't an accurate claim. My eldest cousin was not academically successful. He elected an adolescence of crime with our Uncle Junior, who was three months older, and three months more criminally sophisticated, than my cousin. In the end, my cousin went to prison for bank robbery when I was in the seventh grade. I never saw him again until about ten years ago, when he got out of prison. Then he went back in.

I didn't see him again until last Thanksgiving, when he was out again and telling me about how he'd learned the value of hard work when our older uncles took him to work in the fields. (I remained silent and listened and bit my lip as I struggled not to say, "Weren't you in prison for bank robbery? What hard-work lessons are you talking about?!" I was successful and didn't blurt anything out then.) Shortly after this, we started talking about Latin American literature. He said, "I had a lot of time on my hands, so I read when I was inside." To my great delight, we talked about *One Hundred Years of Solitude.* This is the first time I'd ever been able to talk to anyone in my family about anything academic.

I saw him at his sister's house when he'd been out for a while. I don't know how long. We sat in the apartment living room chatting. He said he'd been sitting in a liquor store parking lot one Sunday morning drinking with some winos. There were four men in all. The one on the end was saying something about his son. My cousin thought, *What's this guy talking about? He's crazy. Already drunk.* Then the guy at the end added that his son was a doctor. Not realizing, until that instant, that this was my genetic father, my cousin interrupted: "Hey, that's my cousin!"

My genetic father was a jazz trumpeter with a heroin habit. A soloist who found possibility in the silence between notes, and during the sound of slurs. I know this from what I hear, because I didn't know him. What did he give me, this father, like other fathers, who give their children things they can touch and things they cannot?

A jazz soloist, say a trumpeter, understands the terrain of silence—both limitation and possibility—before he puts his lips to the mouthpiece. He blows air into the curved tunnels and, through invention and technique, after years of practice, arrives at a singular note that makes the audience vanish into the silences and slurs with him.

That is, if he's any good.

The jazz artist is hero in America: A soloist aware that the individual in democracy, as in a quintet on stage, is, at once, alone, and part of the collective. Jazz is an onomatopoeic version of democracy. Even if the individual is the premier theme of America, the collective, too, matters. This collective is why we stand. At least, it's what we're taught as children—no matter our race.

This erect collective, too, is a matter of American law.

But in medicine, race colors the treatment minority people can expect to receive.

During my speech at a medical conference on race, an audience member asked, "When *does* 'race' apply in medicine?" I rambled on and gave her a vague answer. Until then, I had not read much beneath the skin of race since my days as a rabble-rouser in college. This showed on stage. Then a student from the School of Pharmacy pointed out my speech's intrinsic contradiction: "Dr. Garcia, race is important in pharmacology *because* Blacks metabolize some drugs differently."

Our definitions of race, culture, ethnicity, and the role these words play in American medicine—and all other American places of race, I suspect—differed.

I asked her, "What makes a patient Black?"

What is the "genetic race" of the slave daughter of the master and the slave? The granddaughter's race? The fifth generation? What's the social definition? What's the actual difference?

My language about race missed, entirely, as I answered her question about drug metabolism. I lost the concerned pharmacy student somewhere between miscegenation and the hepatocyte.

And that was before I added a Mexican to the mix!

If I argue in one part of a speech that biological race does not exist, that no nucleotide sequence can portray my race, my linguistic tendencies, my neighborhood, my mother's cooking, my Chinese food preference, my Russian literary leanings, or my easily decipherable American ways, then how can I argue, in another part of that same speech, that race in medicine matters?

Race is important in medicine precisely because of the differences in healthcare that different races of people receive. Alas, racial minorities do not receive inferior healthcare based on race because there's nothing wrong with our race.

Here is where the audience catches me: Race cannot, at once, exist and not exist.

My children are one generation removed from heroin addiction, burglary, robbery, prison, under-education, poverty, beatings, and academic oblivion. Their identities remain suspect in America. Remain liabilities in American medicine.

Race will not disappear. People will ask how she got straight hair, white skin, her interpretation of America. They'll ask this because race can tell them what they want to know about her existence in America. Black people don't ask questions about our children's hair. Black people already know. With curls and color, we can manage on our own. But in medicine, race can make living less likely because of actual medical treatment. Or its absence.

The condition of living in America as a minority has end-organ effects inside of our brown bodies. These biological results can be explained by different biology only sometimes.

I came to America from central California.

When I think of my own entry into the world, I must admit that the role luck played was too great, while democracy took a break, perhaps tired of playing. My mother said, "I think I remember going to the hospital once when I was pregnant with you. I waited to see the doctor, but after six hours, I went home. I didn't even fill the prenatal vitamin prescription the nurse gave me. The next time I went back to the doctor was the night I delivered you."

I wondered what I could have become had I some prenatal vitamins!

I am, at once, a racial minority and a doctor. I titrate my class, education, and knowledge of medicine against the promise of my own poor health based on race.

But my children are growing up with Berkeley-educated parents. A pediatrician, even. They live in a pleasant, safe city and attend top elementary schools. (That education in California is ranked forty-ninth, just above Mississippi, is fodder for another book.)

My children don't need a chapter in a textbook on health disparities to make things better for them. My MD makes things better for them. And I don't suppose I'm talking about other children, either. Rather, as Mae Jemison, MD, the first, the only Black woman astronaut in space, said, "Children aren't our future. We are."

EIGHT

To What End, Diversity?

Donna Elliott

A young African American man, a third-year medical student, had been approached in the library by campus police who were following up on an anonymous report they received about someone in the administration building lobby who "looked as if he didn't belong on campus." The student, a clean-cut, well-dressed, unusually polite, and well-mannered young man, was talking on his cell phone with his father during a rare break from studying medicine. The campus police officers approached him when he returned to the library. (The young man's clean-cut, well-dressed appearance meant nothing when measuring whether he "looked as if" he belonged in medical school.)

The police quickly learned that the young African American man was a medical student and apologized to him for the approach that didn't call into question, but rather answered the question, about his presence in medical school. This reminded me of my own version of reality as a Black medical student thirty-one years ago. In his novel, *Requiem for a Nun*, William Faulkner notes, "The past is never dead. It's not even past."

Was this a story from the 1960s? The 1980s when I was a medical student? No, this event took place in 2010. I understand his experience because of the shared racial experience among Black people in the United States. In essence, and it's not an exaggeration here to say this, the campus police officers had stopped me.

I had originally decided to become a physician because I liked science and was good at it, and because both of my parents grew up during the Depression and took nothing for granted—especially my education. Neither did I. I am a classic baby boomer (you get ahead with hard work and education, I thought). College was to follow high school, in any case. Beyond college: either more education or serious work.

When I was in high school I told my mother, a registered nurse, that I wanted to be a nurse because I liked science and wanted to help people. My mother defined life for me and urged me *not* to become a nurse, but a doctor—more successful, by her definition, than she was. She did not mean that nursing isn't an honorable profession, but rather that I should disregard any artificial limits in life.

Ranked twelfth in my "perfectly" integrated Los Angeles class of seven hundred students, I attended the University of Southern California on a full academic scholarship even after my misguidance counselor pointed me away from college and toward a job. Any little job, I suspect, would have sufficed. In the end, I had no clue, no advice, or no one at all to dissuade me from applying to medical school. (Now, as a dean in the same medical school, USC, I sometimes miss the bliss.)

When I think back and try to remember when I first understood the implications of race, I remember a series of incidents in fifth grade. Another Black girl and I were the only two Black students in a Los Angeles experimental program, unified for fifth and sixth grade. The principal, as part of a conversation on racial issues, asked the otherwise all-White class, "Who would move away if a Black family moved in next door?" The class said they would not. And the principal later said to us, "Isn't that nice that your classmates would not move away?" My friend and I knew something was wrong with the question but could not exactly figure out what. Our mothers, on the other hand, knew exactly what was wrong: It was a case of us and them. Maybe *we* would move away if a White family moved in next door to us. (The teacher never asked.) Our mothers spoke with the principal, made sure she understood the issue, and orchestrated an apology in front of the class.

Later that same year, a mother stood in the doorway open-mouthed when my mother dropped me off at a birthday party. (I have a fair complexion and non-Blacks do not always know I am Black.) After seeing my mother, the woman realized I was Black. In the end, my mother declined to leave me at the party. As a mother, I had the same terrifying insight when my two daughters, ten and twelve, came home from what was to have been a fun adventure with my husband to get ice cream from a local ice cream shop and told me a man in a car yelled and called them "niggers." Ten years later our daughters (one a senior in college, the other a third-year law school student) still feel the shock, the pain, and the reality from that LA summer Saturday incident. Since all incidents are isolated, this one cannot be characterized in that colloquially dismissive manner.

Because of my fifth/sixth-grade experience, along with other experiences, my husband and I, thirty years later, decided *not* to move to a predominantly White area in LA where we could send our children to public school. We bought a house in the upper-middle-class, predominantly Black community, and made the unwise financial commitment to send our daughters to private school, just so we could raise our children with other Black families like ours.

There are two engineers across the street, a business owner next door, a lawyer down the street, two other doctors across the street, and so forth. Our daughters often tell us how they appreciate our unwise financial choice. My eldest daughter recently said that because of who their role models were, it never occurred to her that she would not go to college. They appreciate the constant positive role-modeling they received from our neighbors who became some of our closest friends. Our children learned the same lesson my parents taught me: An intentional lesson. Explicit. Delivered by someone who understands, has experienced, and can chronicle the same reality.

My cousin visited me when I was in medical school. She had been accepted to medical school at both USC and Tulane University. She and I were in the USC gym working out as she tried to decide which school she would attend. A White classmate of mine later asked about my attractive cousin. I innocently thought he might have been romantically interested in her. I explained that she was considering which of the two schools to attend, as she was only in her third year of college, already accepted, and would not need to graduate in order to attend one of these two. He then asked, "What does she have going for her other than being a Black female?"

This question extended to me, naturally. It seemed clear to me that he was asking why *I* was in medical school with *him*, perhaps taking up a spot better suited for a White male, much like him. (I don't know. And don't care to know.) Perhaps he thought I was the recipient of charity or affirmative action, that I did not belong, in any case. I then answered his question for me, not for my cousin—and not for him, I admit. I told him that I would gladly put my GPA, my Medical College Admission Test scores, and my score on any exam we had taken in medical school to date, up against his. While I did not know for sure if I'd win such a comparison, I knew my numbers, I knew the statistics, and I knew the odds were on my side.

My White classmate declined to compare our records.

I remember this day from thirty years ago when someone questioned my value, my competence, my worth, and I knew then, like I know now, that I had something to prove. My parents' words echoed, and still regularly echo, in my head: "In order to get equal recognition for equal work, you cannot produce work of the same quality as your White counterpart. It will have to be better." My parents grew up in the American South, lived through the Depression, took part in the civil rights movement, and created an educated daughter, a doctor, and a medical school dean who is, by all appearances, ensnared in their same historic themes.

I always thought I would have a general pediatrics practice in an underserved Black neighborhood. I had even thought about the exact office. It would be like my own pediatrician's office with a "secret" back-door that children used when they were contagious (or that I used back when I was in college and did not want to be seen in the pediatrician's office). Racial and ethnic minority providers are more likely than their non-minority colleagues to serve in minority and medically underserved communities.[1] Published statistics on minority medical students predicted I'd work there, near my own pediatrician's office. That's also what I predicted I'd do.

I went to USC for medical school, and then trained in the pediatrics residency at the Los Angeles County Hospital in east LA, where I loved the inpatient service. Because I enjoyed the intellectual, the clinical, and the humanity of caring for acutely ill children, I wanted to remain at an academic medical center where I would work on the hospital wards and in the pediatric intensive care unit, where I would teach medical students and residents, and where I would lead clinical research. For the first time, I realized I did not want to be a general pediatrician. I felt as if I were abandoning my destiny and my future patients. I don't mean this question colloquially, or in any way whimsically, but actually: Who would take care of them if I didn't?

An African American male pediatric hematologist was both my mentor and my friend during my residency. He encouraged me to find a way to make a difference in the lives of those same patients in my new path. I wanted to inspire patients, who otherwise would never see a Black physician, strive to make their dreams reality. More than this, I wanted to be the physician for the underserved patients at a large public hospital. I wanted to be in the hub of academic medicine, on the cutting edge of new developments, providing state-of-the-art care.

In my second year as a faculty member, the department chair called me into his office and told me that I would be the new pediatric clerkship director. I had visualized my path as a young clinical scientist. I knew nothing about being a clerkship director beyond having recently completed my pediatrics education and training. The first few years were rough, and then I met a couple of mentors, took some classes in medical education, and let this new intellectual path—medical education—embrace me. Twenty years later, armed with a masters and a doctorate in education, and much experience as a clerkship director, an associate residency program director, and an assistant and associate dean, I recognize that I still have much to do.

As a clinician, educator, and medical school dean, I've made it my job to ensure that all students are treated equally when challenges arise in their education; to provide appropriate mentors for students; and to encourage these students to pursue their academic dreams. Along with others committed to the principle, I've also made it my job to ensure that diversity is understood, valued, appreciated, and embodied. I'm not talking about color diversity here—but actual diversity. The 2002 Institute of Medicine Report, *Unequal Treatment*, notes that increasing the proportion of underrepresented US racial and ethnic minorities among health professionals will allow us, as a country, to place more providers in minority and medically underserved communities. Such an increase is associated with greater patient participation in the care process, higher patient satisfaction, and greater adherence to therapeutic regimens by racial and ethnic minority patients. In short: improved health outcomes.

I encourage minority students to become neurosurgeons, dermatologists, academic physician scientists, and healthcare leaders of the future despite underserved patients' need for primary care physicians, and despite the fact that I, in a way, also abandoned those same patients by choosing academic medicine. I want these young, talented students to hear my mother's message: to not be limited, to be free to disregard any artificial limits. Then how will medical schools make certain that underserved patients have physicians to care for them? We will need to admit more minority students who will return to their neighborhoods; we will need to expose *all students* to underserved patients and teach them how to set aside their biases, to effectively communicate with all patients, even those not like themselves. Especially those.

I currently work with a magnificent White woman whose commitment to underserved patients and communities makes anyone's commitment pale in comparison. She is a family physician who works at a clinic in east LA, joins her patients and others in their work at a community garden, and is the den mother for a Boy Scout troop in South Central Los Angeles.

We can all learn from each other.

The math, however, does not work. We cannot ever educate enough racial minorities to match them with patients in a racially or ethnically balanced way. Nor is this even meaningful. This implies that the Black gastroenterologist in Los Angeles (or lower Alabama, for that matter) should only treat Black people with abdominal pain; that only Russian family practitioners can treat Russians in Sacramento; that an Italo-German cardiologist in Chicago should only treat Italo-Germans with heart disease; and that a Mexican American pediatrician in Arizona should only treat Mexican American children. (What happens when he tries to treat one from Mexico?)

We should appreciate diversity, understand how to teach all physicians to treat all patients, and realize the math runs out quickly in this skin-deep version of how the media portrays diversity. Education about health disparities and cultural competence is now mandated by the medical school accreditation agency. Cultural competence is defined as the ability to recognize and respect diversity of background and opportunity, language, culture, and way of life.[2] Additionally, such education may involve the capacity of providers to effectively identify the health practices and behaviors of diverse populations and to thereby intervene and educate across cultural and language barriers.[3] I worry that in untrained but well meaning hands, cultural competence education can do more harm than good. The last thing we want to do is to perpetuate stereotypes.

Cultural competence education must be about a process to interact with any patient who is different from us. It must be a toolbox, and not a list of "facts" about minority patients or about a particular subset of patients. I wish I'd had such a toolbox in my early practice, where I sometimes worked in an urgent care clinic and came into contact with orthodox Jewish patients. I'm sure my discomfort was palpable. I did not know how to act, what to say, or whom to address. While it is not possible to be completely knowledgeable about all cultures, the awareness that different cultures have different expectations and different rules of appropriate behavior is an important first step for medical schools to teach. All medical schools are required to have a curriculum in cultural competence. Most often the curriculum consists of a few lectures or workshops that all students attend, but the depth of study required to have an impact is often lacking. Cultural competence is not *the* answer to disparities, but turns our attention in that direction. But we must not let that tool diminish the importance of creating a diverse workforce and distract us from the real issues.

I sat in a meeting of medical educators where we discussed the need for increased diversity of faculty. A White PhD male faculty member stated, "Well, you know, there are only a few minority physicians who are qualified to be recruited as faculty." His remark bounced off the walls in the room. Of the fifteen faculty present, four of us were minorities. Even after I had succeeded as a student, a resident, a fellow, a scientist, and a medical school dean, he could only see me as unusual, worth pointing out, and in question. That I have more degrees than he does reminded me of my mother's early warning that I'd have to do more than he would to be able to sit at his table and participate in his discussion. . . . Even a discussion about me.

Racial minority medical students don't have adequate minority faculty to guide, advise, counsel, and remind them of their worth before the campus police approach them, or the campus faculty question their human value. Who will influence academic medical centers, now and in the future, to recruit and train minority students and residents, to develop the science, the policies, and the programs that will increase access to healthcare and reduce diseases that disproportionately afflict minority communities? We need minority physicians who enter medicine specifically to approach their old neighborhoods with the intellect, the training, the point of view, and the humanity required if we are at all serious about closing the gaps among dying Black infants, foot amputations among Mexicans with diabetes, chest pain among Black men, and, let's admit, the inhumanity a minority in medicine can expect from an anonymous call or a procedural question at a faculty meeting questioning her place.

Patients afflicted by healthcare disparities are dependent upon physicians and future physicians who represent their needs. Let's assume each individual doctor attempts to treat each patient correctly. We still face great disparities in both health *care* and health *status*. We need to do more than educate a few minority students in a hostile, or even a welcoming, environment, because the number of such would-be physicians will never be enough. The content also matters. The teachers, themselves, matter.

In medicine, we talk about health outcomes. The outcomes of minority groups could be much better. Having a physician available, going to the physician, believing that your physician has your best interests at heart, and communicating effectively with your physician, along with increasing adherence to prescribed medications and treatments, to recommendations on diet and exercise, are all important factors in decreasing disparities. Can minority doctors, or non-minority doctors who train in an environment with professors from a diverse background, achieve better outcomes? In some respects, the answer is yes. Trust, opportunity, and other numerous factors contribute to healthcare disparities. Patients, social chances, health systems, and doctors likewise contribute. The question remains: To what end, diversity? Race in America is an inextricable, inbred tension in our existence as physicians, medical student educators, and people.

NOTES

1. M. Komaromy, K. Grumbach, et al., "The Role of Black and Hispanic Physicians in Providing Health Care for Underserved Populations," *New England Journal of Medicine* 334, no. 20 (1996): 1305–10.

2. A. Cho, J. Martin, et al., "Incorporating Discussion of Cultural Diversity throughout the First-Year Medical Curriculum," *Journal of the Association of American Medical Colleges* 74, no. 5 (1999): 582–83.

3. J. Zweifler and A. M. Gonzalez, "Teaching Residents to Care for Culturally Diverse Populations," *Academy of Medicine* 73, no. 10 (1998): 1056–61.

NINE

Noblesse Oblige

Jorge A. Girotti

The trip began officially on Holy Thursday, 1974. But the journey had started at least nine years earlier when my dad began convincing some coworkers that the future lay in the United States. My dad did not have much formal education (he was pulled out of school by my grandfather in the eighth grade), but he was a wise person. It was 1965 and, apparently, it was easy then to get a work visa to come to the United States. Several of these individuals went through the process and, within months, were moving to America. Not my dad, though. I guess he felt comfortable in his factory job. By the time he made up his mind, the consulate was reporting a long waiting list. He began the visa application process in 1969, and finally, in late 1973, he was told his file was up for consideration.

By all measures, I had a wonderful childhood. In retrospect, we never had much. We were not deprived of the basics, but we lived *ajustándonos el cinturón* ("tightening our belts") to live within my father's salary. One might describe Virreyes, the Buenos Aires barrio where I grew up, as a lower-middle-class town. About three blocks from our house were a large number of *ranchitos*, modest homes made of the same zinc sheets used for roofing. These contrasts were not a big deal for us. We'd be constantly playing *fútbol* matches against the kids from the *ranchos*, many of whom played barefoot.

My recollection of my first years of schooling is one of a loving, if basic, environment. Before first grade, my godmother Elisa would sit me down next to her (while she mended clothes for a living) to learn how to write numbers and letters; she made me write *palotes* (the capital "I") to get comfortable using a pencil. I walked the ten or so blocks to my school, Escuela N° 21 Juan Bautista Alberti, on my own. Because there weren't many schools, we were assigned to shifts: 8 to 11 a.m., 11 a.m. to 2 p.m., and 2 to 5 p.m. We obviously didn't realize this, but the teachers worked grueling days with full classrooms all day long. I was in the first shift. Since we only had three hours, the teachers kept things at the fundamental level. These women had to love what they did, and as I think about it now, they gave us a great foundation from which to work. I loved our two recesses. Our school had a large interior patio where kids ran around, usually boys playing with other boys, and girls with girls. We all wore knee-length white coats. Some said we wore coats to keep clothes from getting dirty; others said that the coats equalized us so it would not matter what clothes we were wearing.

After eight years at the same school, high school was quite an adventure for me. My dad had made up his mind that I should go to a technical school, Escuelas Técnicas Municipales Raggio, because he felt that getting practical skills was even more important than the diploma. The Raggio school was actually in Buenos Aires, which meant I had a forty-minute train ride from Virreyes to get there. Because students from all over the metro area could apply to the school, everyone had to take placement tests. I took the test for *técnico en publicidad*, or "advertising technician," fully expecting to do very well.

Up to that point I was considered an excellent student and always brought home outstanding report cards. I was devastated to find out I had not passed the test. My dad insisted that we not give up, and that we talk to the school to find out what had happened. Of course, they didn't change the decision, but they told us of another track, *técnico en propaganda*, or "marketing technician," that had low enrollment, and I could just sign up. I did just that. The next five years were exciting and full of promise. I met kids from all over Buenos Aires who became lifelong friends.

During high school, I began writing poetry and short stories and joined a *círculo de niños escritores*, a group of adolescent writers who met once a month to share our work and offer critiques and support. Because the group met downtown, most of the members were from the city. Many came from professional families and were what I considered well-to-do. The woman who directed the group was a sweet, encouraging person who we all guessed had wanted to be an actress: she had a flair for the dramatic. But she was always positive about our writing and made us feel unique and appreciated. I made good friends in this group, different from the people at Raggio, but still light years away from Virreyes.

All through high school I didn't *read* books, but devoured them. My teachers and Maria Emilia (from the writers' *círculo*) would lend me books to take home. It wasn't unusual for me to be reading three books at the same time. I have come to realize that these books, from Argentine to Latin American writers to the Russians to James Joyce and many American greats, shaped my views on life and what we, as individuals, do in the face of good times and bad. As Ernesto Sábato claimed (my paraphrase): A good book is one that has transformed you by the time you are done reading it.

When my dad found out that his visa application was up for consideration, I remember we all sat down around the kitchen table to talk about it. This was late in 1973; free elections had taken place earlier that year. It was not the first time that the military junta had allowed elections. However, it was the first time in over a generation that they agreed to allow a candidate from the *Partido Justicialista*—the party created by Juan D. Perón—to be on the ballot. Not surprisingly, that candidate won by a landslide. There were high expectations that the new president, Héctor José Cámpora, would cede the presidency to Perón, back in Argentina after his eighteen-year exile. This came to pass in June of that year. My dad told my brother and me during our family meeting that he had already lived through Perón's first time in office and didn't want us to go through the same *mierda* ("shit") he had put up with. He knew that the decision to pick up and leave for a foreign culture was a big one for all of us, but he was afraid for the future in Argentina. And so in February 1974, my dad traveled alone to the United States of America. His trip happened just before Carnival—which was a happy, crazy time—and it felt surreal when he told me that, as the oldest, I now was in charge of the house.

The idea was that my dad would go first, hopefully find a job, and rent an apartment, and then my mom, brother, and I would follow. Near the end of the visa process, my dad wrote to three guys who had moved to the United States. One he knew from the factory; he and his family lived in Boston. The second one was my godmother's brother, who lived in Philadelphia. The third was my godfather's brother-in-law, who had moved to the Chicago area. Maybe it was fate that the only response came from the couple in Chicago, saying they would be happy to help while he settled down. These people lived in Highland Park, a suburb thirty miles north of Chicago. Through them my dad met another Argentine who was a carpenter and was able to get my dad a job in a shop specializing in custom wood flooring in the North Shore.

With my dad now settled in the United States, we decided it was time for my mom, brother, and me to go. We made the arrangements to travel in April. As the day of my trip got closer, all kinds of emotions flooded me. It was at once exciting, scary, and sad to know I would soon leave behind all the people who had made me who I was. Our itinerary took us to Rio de Janeiro for a quick stop, then on to New York's Kennedy Airport, and finally to Chicago. That early morning arrival in New York was a brutal reminder that I didn't know as much English as I thought. After we cleared customs and immigration, it was up to me to get us to the next plane. When I tried my broken, cryptic English to ask for directions, well-intentioned *gringos* would speak a string of syllables in what seemed like a single, mile-long word. Lucky for us, we came across Spanish-speaking folks who pointed us to the right place. We got to Chicago on Good Friday. Coming out of the airport and to our ride to Highland Park, the air felt chilly. I was shocked to see people in shorts and flip-flops and thought everyone had gone mad. It was only after my first full year in the area that I came to appreciate what April's air feels like after a Midwest winter.

I was advised to start taking English as a Second Language (ESL) classes that were offered for free at a community college in Waukegan. Having read most of Ray Bradbury's books, I thought it was amazing that I was now learning English in his hometown. My typical routine included taking classes in the morning and then working the second shift for ServiceMaster, cleaning offices all over the north suburbs. I do remember, as my English skills improved, having to go with my mom or dad to doctor visits to interpret for them. This felt very strange, since in Argentina I was totally clueless about my parents' health. It was particularly awkward to be in the middle when my mom saw a doctor. I had to translate sensitive information and learned of issues that perhaps a son should not know about his mother.

By the summer of 1975 my ESL teacher (a sweet, Scandinavian woman named Anika Stefansen) was sure she could not teach me any more than what I already knew. She pushed me to register at the main campus of the College of Lake County and take college courses. Earlier that summer I had found a job at Abbott Labs in North Chicago, working in the IV packaging line. Most of my coworkers were Latinos, from either Mexico or Puerto Rico. My supervisor noticed that I spoke Spanish and had decent English skills. Just before I was to start the fall semester, the company offered to make me a line supervisor in the first shift with a sizable raise. I don't know exactly why, but I decided to turn down the offer and quit work to study full-time.

School was a lot of fun, even though I was a bit older and had an accent. I was enjoying my classes. In one of my art classes I met Joe Montain. Joe wanted to be a graphic designer, and I learned he was planning to transfer to a four-year university. We became very good friends, going out every weekend and hanging out on school days. Joe lived in the far northwest suburbs with his dad; his mom had passed away when he was young. As the time to apply to universities got nearer, Joe said we should go visit these places. So we set out to visit our two main choices: Illinois State University and the University of Illinois at Urbana-Champaign. I had no clue of what to look for. We were admitted to both universities and chose the latter, so, in the fall of 1977, I moved to Champaign to live with Joe and Warren, a Vietnam veteran we had met at school.

Moving away from home—this time from my own family—was a traumatic experience for all of us. I had become the "liaison" between my parents and the outside world. My younger brother was more independent and didn't particularly like being the go-between. My dad had quit working at the flooring shop and was repairing antique furniture on his own. I'd go with him to clients' homes to give estimates and move furniture back and forth. Leaving home was hard, and my parents were not convinced that more schooling would do me any good. But I left.

I moved back home two years later, now with a bachelor's degree and aiming to be an art teacher. Having lived with Americans for so long, I didn't realize how difficult it was to get back into Spanish; my mom would joke that I had become mute. I started using Spanglish, and even my Spanish wasn't that Argentine anymore, as I'd met a number of Latin Americans from all over the continent and picked up words from different regions.

Finding a teaching position proved to be more difficult than I anticipated. Apparently there weren't that many positions for recently graduated, inexperienced teachers. Through friends of my parents, I learned of a counseling position at Aspira of Illinois, a community agency in Waukegan. My job would be to encourage young people in high school to consider careers in healthcare. I knew nothing about counseling, and even less about healthcare (except that it was hard when your doctor didn't speak your language). But this was a full-time job and I could start making money. So, in March 1980, I became a counselor.

The job at Aspira taught me a lot about what it means to be Hispanic in the United States. It taught me even more about what it's like to be brown in this country. I dealt with teachers and counselors at the local high schools, where I tried to get permission to contact Hispanic students who showed promise in science and math and introduce them to the wide array of healthcare careers. They thought that these students would not cut it in those fields and, after all, it would be unfair to offer extra resources to some students and not others. The doors were closed on reaching out to students in the high schools. There was no way I could meet the agency's expectations for the number of contacts and participants I was supposed to have in the program.

By December of that year, it was clear that the program would not work in Waukegan. The director then decided to bring me to the Chicago office to expand the healthcare careers program there. The Chicago office was nothing like Waukegan; things were actually happening there. My colleague, Robert Martinez, had built a wonderful program to expose college students to medicine and other health fields. He told me he would enjoy working with high-school-level students more, and wanted me to take over the college component.

This job was a transition point for me. I began to grasp the pragmatic realities of making a living in something other than art. It also opened my eyes in a big way again to the realities of what it meant to grow up Hispanic in the United States. Growing up in Argentina, the clearest discrimination you could feel was based on socioeconomic standing. While Argentines come from a variety of backgrounds—Western and Eastern European, Asians, Middle Easterners, Native peoples, and so on—I never felt that "color lines" meant anything. However, I could feel a palpable difference along "money lines." If there was ever any external-ly or internally imposed barrier to my dreams, it was built on the fact that we came from poverty.

But in the United States, I began to realize that ethnicity had a lot to do with your prospects, above and beyond what your socioeconomic stand-ing might be. Unquestionably, these two factors intersect so often that it's hard to see where the lines begin and end. In other words, most students I met were Hispanic *and* poor. In order to succeed, they had to overcome elements they didn't control. I had always rooted for the underdog; the job at Aspira introduced me to many young men and women who were achieving against all odds. I began to develop a sense of mission with broader implications than teaching arts to youngsters. I didn't know much at all about medicine or any other health profession, but they ap-peared to be noble ways to give back and serve a real need.

In 1981 I met someone who, in many ways, set my professional path: Bob Walker. Bob had just arrived at the University of Illinois College of Medicine to direct a relatively new initiative called the Urban Health Program (UHP). He was a New Yorker and had studied and worked in New York, Washington, DC, and Boston-area universities. Bob was Black but seemed to have a clearer vision for the need to diversify the work-force beyond Blacks. Over the next year and a half, we collaborated on many activities to expose my students to medicine and U of I. In the late spring of 1982, Bob called to tell me his assistant was leaving, and he wanted me to apply for the job. I was genuinely enjoying my work at Aspira, but the possibility of a job on "hard money" (i.e., funded through a recurring budget instead of short-term grants) with better benefits was difficult to resist. My colleagues also said that my impact would be great-er by working at the university. When I broke the news to Aspira's direc-tor, he was obviously not thrilled, but said he was happy for me for the opportunity.

And so, in October 1982, the next phase of my career began at U of I. Bob made it clear what he wanted: higher numbers and a more diverse group of minority students. That fall the college had enrolled seventy-five minority students; the following year the number went up to ninety-five out of 331. Bob was very happy, but not everyone in the college shared his joy. The university had never seen this level of enrollment for a group that was clearly nontraditional. In retrospect, it is easy to see that we were not ready for the kind of needs these students would bring with them. To complicate things, the faculty, in general, was not necessarily well suited for teaching a diverse classroom. When many students began to fail in the curriculum, the faculty naturally put the blame on the students.

For the rest of the decade, enrollment of minority students remained high (though never again at ninety-five). But so did our rate of attrition. At the time, I felt that this was "just the way things were": high attrition was the price to pay to expand inclusion. It is true that for every case that ended with a student's dismissal, another student with the same credentials made it through. It must be that those intangible qualities could not be accurately assessed at the time of application—to tease out who would succeed and who would not.

In 1984, at Bob Walker's strong suggestion, I began my PhD studies in the College of Education. Bob's logic made sense: If you like working in academia, you need their union card—the doctorate. I am sure I didn't know what I was getting into, but I found the courses made a lot of sense with the day-to-day reality I saw in my job. I would not have finished the doctoral degree had it not been for my wife's support. Between work and school, it was not easy putting up with me. By the time I completed all of the course work and passed the preliminary examination, we had two children (Jorge Luis and Marjorie) and had bought our first home. It took a while to figure out what to write for my thesis, but I finally settled on a qualitative study of socialization into the physician role of minority medical students. As with most graduate students, I wanted the "perfect" thesis, and kept tinkering with the chapters and adding to the bibliography. I was afraid to turn in my work to my adviser for fear of being shot down. My wife once again brought me back to reality, lovingly letting me know I would end up without a family unless I turned in my draft thesis right away. Of course, I did. My adviser thought it was ready for defense, and I completed my doctorate in 1990. By then I had lost my dad to a massive heart attack. I am not sure he would have approved anyway, since, in his mind, any education after high school didn't make much sense.

Suddenly I became "Doctor Girotti." I could now claim expertise in one particular area of knowledge. Within the next year, three important things happened in the professional realm: I was named assistant dean, was selected from a national pool of candidates for the prestigious fellowship sponsored by the American Council on Education (ACE), and received my first federal grant as principal investigator for the Hispanic Center of Excellence (HCOE). These were momentous events for me, and from each I learned invaluable lessons.

The assistant dean position meant more work in areas other than minority affairs. Again, with Bob's mentorship, I ventured into issues in general student affairs, dealing with the dean's letters and the residency match process for graduating medical students. In the yearlong ACE fellowship, I met some amazing individuals from all over the country and learned the highs and lows of higher administration. A clear goal of the fellowship was to nurture future college presidents. However, I learned that (at least at that time) I did not want to be a college president. The HCOE grant opened another national network for me, one that I still treasure today. It also sharpened my ability to create and maintain budgets and systematically evaluate programs. As the 1990s progressed, I became more confident in my ability to lead and learned that my style was not confrontational, but collaborative. I tried to make my case with evidence, but I was still trying to sharpen the nature of the evidence. What is the benefit of increasing ethnic and racial diversity in medicine? What are the elements that make the case a win-win proposition? We had *Bakke* (the Supreme Court split decision on affirmative action), but its pillars were sagging just as the number of applicants to medical schools was reaching record proportions.

The year 1994 started on a very auspicious note. Once again Bob Walker was helping to open doors for me. The dean, trying to quell internal dissension, moved one person and made me director of admissions for the College of Medicine. At that time, I had been working with the admissions staff for a while because my minority recruitment activities intersected significantly with that office. Everyone there felt that the previous director was constantly looking over their shoulders and not trusting their professional skills. My approach was to have mutually agreeable work outcomes and let staff do their jobs without micromanaging their time. I didn't even move into the same office in an effort to give them their space.

In October of that year, two major events took place: My daughter Daniela was born and, on the same day, I learned that Bob was leaving the college. I still don't know exactly what led to his resignation, but do know that his health had taken a turn for the worse. Bob told me when he called to congratulate us on our new baby. After twelve years of working together, the news hit me hard. Bob had been the big brother I never had. In his phone call, he mentioned he had recommended to the dean that I become the director of the UHP. I was ecstatic and scared: I would be the first non-Black to direct UHP.

The sheer magnitude of what we were trying to do struck me. This was not just an admissions mandate. We were responsible for educating and graduating competent doctors. Could we justify having 15–18 percent attrition rates as a price of doing business? The next year represented a unique opportunity to make a mark—to see if two seemingly disparate goals could be reconciled: maintain high admissions numbers and significantly increase graduation. The first area I focused on was the nature of our support system. Minority students had told me that the academic support system we had did not address their needs. I had to fire the person in charge and restructure how we did things. This meant creating a new position for an academic skills specialist. It also meant doing a better job of identifying students who needed our services the most.

One of the challenges I confronted was that the college didn't have support services for the general student body. This fact led to many tensions about resources and what students perceived as "privileges." We devised a mechanism to identify and "enroll" students into support services based on need rather than ethnic/racial background. This meant that some majority students were invited and some minority students were not. Given our history, this was a risky proposition.

The next initiative focused on better understanding the qualities— academic and personal—that led to success. To that end, I recommended to the admissions committee that we institute conditional admissions. We started this approach with two students for the entering class of 1996. They were mandated to take and pass a six-week Summer Prematriculation Program (SPP) that previewed the first semester of medical school. We had had this program for many years, but participation was open to all admitted minority students on a first-come, first-served basis. This change would mean that candidates mandated by the committee to successfully complete the SPP would have priority over regularly admitted applicants. The first two students successfully completed both the program and the MD degree in four years. The following year, we applied for supplemental funds through the Health Careers Opportunity Program (HCOP) to establish a post-baccalaureate admissions program; the program began in 1997. These students also were offered conditional admissions but had to successfully complete a fourteen-month program.

By 1999, as we got better at the selection process and the provision of support services, our attrition rate dropped to 5 percent. In the process of identifying student needs, I learned an important lesson: The UHP was based on the premise that minority individuals would want to serve minority patients in minority communities. I learned that a good number of them did not want to do that. They had a different vision for their future. I remember asking students, "If you had to sign a pledge that you would pursue that particular path, would you do it?" The group was evenly divided. This lesson became critical for me a few years later as I tried to wrestle with ways to improve career choices focused on under-served urban communities.

Things seemed to be going well, but problems were brewing. After more internal dissension—and one week before 9/11—I resigned my post as director of UHP. It had been a productive nineteen-year ride, but it was time to move on. I became dean of Special Curricular Programs, an umbrella that brought together our baccalaureate-MD and joint degrees with public health and business administration (MD/MPH, MD/MBA). It also opened the door to develop a new curricular offering: the Urban Medicine (UMed) curriculum. This curriculum begins with the premise that to make an impact on the availability of physicians in underserved urban communities, at least two things have to happen: Participants have to be properly selected at entry—not based on their ethnic/racial back-grounds, but on their track record—and they have to be nurtured throughout medical school.

This was not a novel idea; several analogous rural health programs had demonstrated its effectiveness. However, the evidence for urban set-tings was not as clear. For the next two years, we looked for someone to fund this concept on a pilot basis. We went to local and national founda-tions, federal agencies, and so forth. Everyone loved the concept, but no one was funding those particular initiatives. In the fall of 2004, my boss said, "Let's just do this." In 2005, we enrolled the first cohort of twelve UMed students. That same year the dean gave us a small budget that allowed us to hire an assistant director and a graduate assistant. For fall 2006, we doubled the cohort size to twenty-four students. The UMed has evolved dramatically since its inception; nowadays we typically have over one hundred applicants per year. They are active in all college and community activities and get involved in progressive organizations, speaking up more often about issues that they perceive as affecting students and patients.

For the past two years, the Chicago Community Trust, a local foundation that supports a variety of initiatives, has provided funding for UMed. Currently, the program carefully selects participants from those admitted to the college. Candidates must make a separate application to the program. Upon entry, students take part in a longitudinal, four-year curriculum that consists of interactive didactic sessions built on four themes: community, health disparities, cross-cultural clinical skills, and leadership and advocacy. The curriculum is presented in "spiral" fashion, returning each year to revisit topics from a different perspective that build on previous learning. We have begun development of a supplemental web-based curriculum on each major topic to serve as an additional resource for students.

In addition to the didactic component, students must complete a Longitudinal Community Rotation (LCR), which begins in the first year and concludes in the fourth year. Students work in small teams (three or four students each) with community partners in an effort to develop community-based solutions to promote health or prevent disease. Partners may be community clinics or social service agencies; however, we expect UMed students' work will be of a non-clinical nature, since other components of the curriculum already address that issue. Ideally, we expect that as students move on with their education, other UMed students can continue the partnership to either sustain existing projects or develop new ones. Each student must log a minimum of two hundred hours in the LCR, and at the end the team turns in a final paper, which can be one of the following: (a) an evaluation of a particular program, (b) a proposal for funding the selected program or its next logical continuation, or (c) a traditional research paper.

We have learned several important lessons. Women are much more likely than men to identify with the program's mission. There is a strong interest from minority students, *but* other groups also share a genuine commitment to the plight of urban residents, the majority of whom are poor and of minority background. It is too early to tell if this chapter's title makes sense, at least if we focus on the Urban Medicine curriculum as one approach to improve healthcare quality and availability in urban settings. Does, in fact, nobility oblige those from privileged backgrounds to serve and give back to the disenfranchised in our society? Is the fact that those individuals do not need to worry about their skin color an insurmountable barrier to ethnic/racial divides? Are we better off directing minority students into this pathway because they literally have skin in the game?

It will take more time to begin to see the impact of the Urban Medicine curriculum. To date we have had three classes of UMed graduates (2009–2011). As a group, they are selecting primary care fields (family medicine, internal medicine, obstetrics/gynecology, and pediatrics) at a higher rate than their counterparts. However, the desirable outcomes of the program—practitioner, researcher, advocate, and policymaker—are not necessarily tied to specific medical specialties, and they certainly may not become apparent during residency training. In the meantime, we continue to sharpen the focus of the curriculum so that participants see the added value to all the extra work right away.

In the end, it may be argued that the health of the public is everyone's responsibility. This should matter to everyone because we are, in fact, all in it together. It is our responsibility to engage younger generations in this critical goal. All patients deserve access; all patients deserve physicians who care, who will put their skins, whatever color they may be, in the game for their patients. At stake is the health of the nation.

TEN

In France, Once

Myrtis Sullivan

I grew up in racially segregated south Chicago—the same Chicago that Lorraine Hansberry portrayed in her classic play, *A Raisin in the Sun* (1959). During my preteen years, I began to understand that things were different for Whites and Blacks. But I didn't know the details of these differences in education, law enforcement, housing, and so forth. I lived in a lower-middle-class (or upper-lower-class) neighborhood. It was understood, somehow, passively, that we could not cross the boundary streets of our Black neighborhood into the adjacent White one. Black children were regularly cautioned about "crossing the line" that divided these communities. In the 1960s, our neighborhoods were segregated, but relatively safe. Our schools were overcrowded, but we had great teachers. Most families in my neighborhood were headed by parents or grandparents who were poor, but very proud, people who had come to Chicago from the Deep South during the Great Migration.

Just as in Hansberry's play, most of these former migrants had their dreams deferred, or denied, but still worked hard to try to make a better life for their children and grandchildren. They were domestics, factory and construction workers, dishwashers, cooks and waiters, and the like. The neighborhood was segregated, but some Black white-collar workers and educators also lived there. Although some Blacks owned corner grocery stores, most of the businesses in our neighborhood were owned by Whites.

The American Institute for Foreign Study awarded me a scholarship to study French in Vichy, France, during the summer before my junior year in high school. There was only one other Black student, who had also received a scholarship, among the dozens of students in the group to which I was assigned. The rest of the group was made up of White students from Rhode Island and Pittsburgh. The group was further divided into smaller units, and the girls and boys lived in separate dormitories. So I rarely interacted with the other Black student, a young man. We studied in Vichy, took weekend excursions to Paris and Geneva, and spent a week in London.

Traveling to Europe was life-changing for me: I saw cities and landmarks I'd read about throughout elementary and junior high school. While exciting and unique, this experience also left me feeling homesick, alone, and isolated. The girls in the group were very friendly; I was not mistreated at all. However, I encountered daily reminders of how different I was from everyone else. Some of the reminders were my dark skin color, my hair texture, my background—inner-city low income as compared with mostly wealthy White girls. I was frequently asked, "Why are you so shy and quiet?" and "Do you have an Afro?" After a few weeks in Vichy, my loneliness and homesickness intensified. I withdrew from the group and began to spend most of my time alone. I started reading more, and writing letters to my family and friends back home in Chicago.

One of the adult chaperones gave me a book, *The Autobiography of Malcolm X*, which I read in its entirety. I had never heard of Malcolm X and was not aware of the emerging Black Power and Black Is Beautiful movements. After talking with the chaperone and reading the autobiography, I began to realize that although I was from the segregated south side of Chicago, I was proud of the rich heritage of my ancestors who sacrificed their lives during slavery, and beyond, in America. I began to consider that I, too, had a responsibility to contribute to the rich legacy I had inherited.

During that summer, I also got a chance to visit Switzerland and England; I was able to see and appreciate a world that existed beyond my neighborhood and my hometown. Spending time with the other youth in my group, my eyes were opened to the physical, cultural, financial, and educational differences and disparities that existed among Black and White Americans. After reading *The Autobiography of Malcolm X*, I learned what he meant by "Black pride" and "Black power," and I began to feel that I had a responsibility to address the injustices about which he spoke in his book: "I am a human being first and foremost, and as such I'm for whoever and whatever benefits humanity as a whole."

I was struck by the contrasts between Europe and Chicago. I was amazed by the number of Blacks I saw in Paris. There were dark-skinned young men sitting in sidewalk cafés; occasionally I saw Blacks in the hotels we visited in France and Switzerland. I later found out that most of the Blacks I encountered in France and Switzerland did not speak English. Most of them were probably from Africa. I think I was so shocked to see them because I had never seen that many Blacks in downtown Chicago. In my segregated neighborhood, we rarely saw White people strolling about, aside from the occasional salesmen and shop owners. Our churches, schools, and parks were all segregated. And during the mid-1960s, few Blacks were on television.

Blacks appeared to be able to move around more freely in Paris and the other places I visited. Before I visited Europe, I could not recognize a world beyond segregated south Chicago. In France, once I realized that I was lonely and homesick—like any other teenager away anywhere for an entire summer—and separated myself from the rest of the students, I understood that I was isolated in America, my home.

The next summer, before my senior year in high school, I accepted a summer job through the Urban League. They assigned me to an affluent hospital in downtown Chicago. In the course of my duties, I discovered that the hospital employed only one Black physician. I found this ordinary version of reality perplexing at first, and then, after a few days, shocking. I had wanted to become a teacher or a criminal defense attorney prior to working at the White hospital. But as I examined my own reasons for these two options—either education or law—I considered becoming a doctor. Insofar as I'd thought of the other two possibilities as ways to help people in my neighborhood—or ones like it, let's say— I wondered if I could find a life inside medicine itself where I might help.

I attended a small liberal arts college in Illinois mainly because an alumnus recruited me. My mantra throughout college was, *Give back to my community*. Give what it gave me: self-confidence, a belief that I could accomplish anything for which I worked, a sense of pride, and the hope of helping people less fortunate. My friends at Illinois Wesleyan University thought my ferocity was both compelling and amusing. Whenever I thought about changing my major from biology/pre-med to French (my favorite subject) and giving up on medicine entirely during the tough college years, these amused friends used my mantra against me and reminded me that I *must* become a doctor and "give back to my community." I suspect they also felt it was important to them, and ultimately to the community itself, that they support me, the only Black pre-med student in our class at our small, isolated, historically and predominantly White liberal arts college.

After graduating from IWU, I went back to Chicago, where I attended medical school. I was both fortunate and determined. The future was upon me. My medical school class was approximately 9 percent women and 10 percent minority (Black and Hispanic). Most of the Black students banded together to form study groups. Unfortunately, a number of students did not survive the rigorous exams and other stressors of those four years. Still others survived, but had to repeat one or two years because they'd failed exams or clinical rotations. The feeling of isolation I felt earlier in life returned during my clinical rotations. One incident during my internal medicine rotation at an upscale hospital on the north side of Chicago was particularly upsetting. I was on morning rounds with the attending physician and a group of three White male medical students. We walked into the room of a White female patient. Before the attending started to check on the patient, she told him that she wanted to speak to him alone.

He asked us medical students to leave the room, spoke with her, then came to retrieve us a few minutes later. The patient had told him that she did not want me in her room. He'd told her that none of the students would come if the entire team could not accompany him. So the entire group walked back into the room and observed the attending's interaction with his patient. While I felt grateful and appreciated his support and defense, the entire incident was difficult for me. Embarrassing, frustrating, humiliating. I felt different, isolated from the group.

Medical school was very challenging and emotionally draining. But with hard work, support from my Black peers and older students, and resources from the Minority Opportunity Program (nicknamed "MOP"), I survived. I chose to train in pediatrics at Cook County Hospital. I felt County would be an oasis compared to the other hospitals I knew from my third and fourth years of medical school. Their staffs were predominantly White, and the hospitals had nearly no Black or Hispanic patients.

While I felt much more comfortable working with minority patients and a diverse clinical and support staff, Cook County Hospital was not the oasis I had envisioned. Unexpected racism and isolation again reared their ugly heads. Five of the eighteen interns were Black. This was a great comfort at first. However, we soon began to share stories about actual (or perceived) incidents in which we were treated unfairly or differently from the other residents. A few of my Black colleagues reported that they were constantly berated while on rounds, or told that their work was not up to par. We also learned of several occasions when some of the White residents were invited to the homes of attending physicians, while we were not. The attendings were constantly getting the names of the Black residents wrong or mixed up. This feeling of discrimination culminated in three of the five Black residents leaving the program. Only two of us were left to finish.

I decided to stay because I loved my patients and the camaraderie of the other Black residents at County in other specialty training programs. I knew conditions were not optimal, but still thought that Cook County was probably better than some of the other programs because of the clinical experience I could gain and the diversity of the staff and patient population.

After residency I was accepted into the Ambulatory Pediatrics Fellowship program at County. This gave me an opportunity for additional training in the outpatient clinics and emergency room, as well as the chance to complete the master's program at the School of Public Health at the University of Illinois at Chicago, where I chose to specialize in maternal-child health. While working on the front line at County, I had begun to see how social isolation and racial and financial inequities manifested themselves in the inner city. Low immunization rates led to measles and whooping cough epidemics among Black and Hispanic toddlers. Crime, violence (domestic and neighborhood), teen pregnancy, and sexually transmitted infections were rampant.

I continued to work in that immense public hospital in Chicago as an emergency medicine pediatrician for over two decades—first as a staff pediatrician, and ultimately as the chief of pediatric emergency medicine. These were my two decades of "giving back." My own personal experience is an example of why there is national focus on increasing diversity in the health professions. According to the Sullivan Report (no relation to me!), increasing diversity means that minority professionals are more likely to serve minority and medically underserved populations, and increased diversity among physicians would likely "improve the overall health of the nation . . . [the entire US population] will benefit from a health workforce that is culturally sensitive and focused on patient care."[1]

Despite the severe minority underrepresentation, Cook County's residents, attending staff, and support staff were perhaps the most diverse in the city during my residency, and later as a supervising attending. But, in fact, as of 2015, in the more than one hundred years of the hospital's existence, there have been only two Black chairpersons in obstetrics/gynecology, two in family medicine, and one very short-lived chair of pediatrics. There has been only one Hispanic. There has never been a Black or Hispanic chair of internal medicine, emergency medicine, psychiatry, or surgery.

With the severe primary care physician shortages, the antiquated public hospital system where I worked for decades still promises long waits for patients in the ER and in the pharmacy. Families travel significant distances on buses or elevated trains, often with several young children in tow, only to wait. For those who are fortunate enough to have cars, parking is insufficient. The parking lots are often filled beyond capacity by physicians and hospital employees with parking privileges, requiring families to park in a public lot located a half mile away, or to search for a parking meter. When families finally arrive at the clinic, they can expect to be treated rudely, and sometimes—if they are late to one of the clinics due to the aforementioned inconveniences and hassles, or any of the other daily challenges of being poor—they may even be turned away without being examined by a doctor.

I was struck by the way communication across cultures can play an important role in health outcomes. It often requires doctors to first listen to understand their patients, and then act. If patients' concerns or needs are not fully understood or addressed, health outcomes can be adversely affected.

I offer two examples. In the first, what may seem to be a simple language barrier ultimately also illustrates how inadequate communication can result in physicians and other healthcare providers' failure to understand how people interpret illness, and how the way they use the healthcare system can result in delay of treatment. The second example demonstrates the power of supporting a young Black mother, and how listening to her and understanding her concerns and needs can help ensure the best outcome for her pregnancy because we know the impact of social determinants on health outcomes.

A four-year-old Mexican American boy's parents complained of the child's vague abdominal pain and a rash on his arms. They had visited family and friends in Mexico a few weeks prior to bringing him to the Continuity Clinic for a check-up. After a thorough physical exam and lengthy discussion with the family about the boy's condition with the assistance of a Spanish interpreter, I sent them home with instructions to collect stool specimens. In order to collect the stool sample, the family was given two small bottles filled with a solution and were told to bring the solution back to the clinic in one week so we could send the stool sample to the laboratory for analysis. The family returned to the clinic without the bottles. I asked the interpreter to ask the family why they returned without the stool sample. After an animated discussion with the family, the interpreter turned to me and said, "The family did not understand the instructions we gave them. Instead of collecting a stool sample and placing it in the solution, they applied the solution to their son's rash."

The second example involves a young African American woman who had just learned that she was pregnant again when she gave a testimony at our Maternal and Infant Mortality Summit. Devastated by the loss of her twins the previous year, she was determined that this second pregnancy would be successful. She vowed to be more assertive and more diligent about her prenatal care. She expressed anger at the doctors she had blindly trusted to care for the twins. Her anger was directed at the doctors, and at herself, for losing the twins. She understood that twins could be more difficult than a single birth, so she had tried to do everything right—kept scheduled appointments, eaten responsibly, taken prenatal vitamins, not overexerted herself. When she began experiencing problems, she worried and asked her doctor if she could be referred to a high-risk perinatologist. Her doctor told her that this wasn't necessary.

Perhaps it wasn't. Perhaps her twins would not have survived in any case. But she felt the healthcare system had failed her, did not listen to her when she tried to alert her doctor that she feared something had gone wrong with her pregnancy.

These two examples, for me, show that we still have work to do to improve quality and access to care for underserved groups. While programs like All-Kids (Illinois's Medicaid program that provides universal health insurance coverage for all infants, children, and adolescents to age twenty-one) and the new federal Affordable Care Act have great potential to drastically improve health and healthcare, currently unacceptable disparities in health outcomes persist—particularly with infant mortality, cardiovascular disease, and cancer.

According to the Centers for Disease Control, a Black infant in the United States is two and a half times more likely to die when compared with an analogous White infant. Inner-city Black and Latino children live (and die) with worse asthma, and they use preventive asthma medication less often than White children within the same managed care populations. In addition, minority children with asthma are more likely to be hospitalized.

If (and when) the Affordable Care Act is fully operational, we will need even more primary care physicians and other health professionals on the front lines in cities like Chicago, New York, Dallas, Los Angeles, and the like. If they do not come through the cities' population pipelines, we will have to import them from abroad, as was done in the 1950s and 1960s. According to the Sullivan Report, the "ghosts of segregation [and discrimination] continue to haunt."[2] These ghosts need not rear their ugly heads. A singular trip to France changed my life. My journey through the educational and career pipeline is a testament to the realm of possibilities and opportunities for all African American and Hispanic youth.

NOTES

1. The Sullivan Commission, *Missing Persons: Minorities in the Health Professions. A Report of the Sullivan Commission on Diversity in the Healthcare Workforce*, 2004, http://www.aacn.nche.edu/media-relations/SullivanReport.pdf, 3.
2. Ibid., 5.

Part IV

Toward Solutions

Aristotle's discussion of forensic discourse in *The Art of Rhetoric* attempts to persuade the audience to see things differently—better. Race in medicine is a branch of race in America, and it cannot be left totally in the hands of physicians, independent of the other institutions' contributions. We are not proposing to right any wrongs, per se. A substantive national discussion will allow the dissonance and encourage the natural collaborative discourse promised by this varied group of writers in concert with the audience. The audience here, like the audience in a jazz club, is actually a required part of the "discussion." The speakers, and what they have to say, remain anemic without a serious audience "participating" in this exchange.

ELEVEN

The Nisei Veteran Played the Ukulele

Sylvia Gates Carlisle

I sat on the Brown University medical school admissions committee as a student. The standard introduction on applicants' personal essays was "I like science and want to help people." Until that point I never realized how many people liked science and wanted to help people. It turns out that *all* applicants claim these two attributes on the way to becoming a doctor. At Brown we prided ourselves on treating each medical school candidate as an individual, and assigned two committee members to review each application. Even though Brown marketed its multifaceted diversity, in each of the two years I sat on the admissions committee we faced two thousand impressively similar applications from people who were not just inanimate numbers or packets of information.

Before I understood medical school admissions from the inside, I suspect that, in most ways, I was just like these homogeneous applicants. I lacked a clear understanding of what I passionately pursued—the eternal pre-medical conundrum. How will I know what I want to do with my life before starting the eleven years of education and training—eleven years *after* I'd chosen that irrevocable career path?

I found that my classmates who were doctors' children enjoyed an understanding of the operations of medical practice. Even among their applications, however, I found few personal essays that shone through the dross. Hardworking and intelligent, certainly. Necessary, but not sufficient to create a good doctor. We didn't have to worry about dumb, lazy people becoming doctors. With sixty-two seats, give or take, and limited information about the person the application represented, sifting through the similarities to find the kernels of uniqueness that differentiated one from the other became the first priority. As a school that recruited nontraditional students, we had some relief from all of the enthusiastic biology majors with good grades, good test scores, and some volunteer work.

But what makes a great doctor? Are they born or nurtured? In the post-*Baake* era, schools obsessed over test scores and GPAs while recognizing that these numbers only predicted first-year performance, not graduation rates. Not ethics. Not competence. I'd want a surgeon to have good hand-eye coordination, but the application process fails to uncover that skill. Facing a life-threatening disease, I'd want empathy, not a brilliant robot. Television's Dr. House might make the diagnosis, but could he help a real person successfully fight a disease? We excavated, trying to uncover the critical unmeasureables: compassion, self-awareness, integrity. I had used the common superficial narrative in my own admissions essay, but was accepted to medical school in spite of what I'd written, which, as I realize now, must have sounded much like the others. Maybe the admissions committee saw something I had unknowingly articulated.

My mother tells me that I wanted to be a doctor, and not a nurse, from the time before I can remember. I wanted to listen to a heart and make someone better. How does a Black girl growing up in Portland, Oregon, in the 1960s decide to be a doctor? I knew TV's *Julia*, played by the elegant Diahann Carroll, was a nurse. *Marcus Welby, MD*, played by the stereotypically fatherly Robert Young, was not a possibility for me, but I had made up my mind. Guidance counselors notwithstanding, I saw myself doctoring people Black like me. They saw a young, completely unrealistic dreamer. The last Black student in the college-prep track at my high school was three years my senior. But my parents were part of the generation from the Jim Crow South, groomed in Black colleges to be "ready for integration." That meant working to be prepared when the window of opportunity cracked open. Their professors demanded excellence. And their parents instilled both excellence and a dedication to service that my parents continued. Daddy's best friend, a general practice doctor serving the Black community in Portland, might have been a beacon, but we were his friends, not his patients. He and Daddy shared season tickets to the Portland Trailblazers. I think the biggest factor in my choice to become a physician was the importance my parents placed on service, which they learned from their own parents, who'd grown up during Reconstruction. (My paternal grandfather, John Wesley Gates, was born in 1864 and, after his wife died, raised eleven children and cared for his parents. He owned one hundred acres and joined a small contingent of tough and mean independent Black farmers who kept land for years despite Mississippi violence that persisted through the 1960s. His children, including my father, spent years in activism and volunteerism. My maternal grandfather, James Gordon McPherson, was born in 1873. Returning with the 24th Infantry from San Juan Hill, he had the nerve to expect equal treatment, earning the right for Blacks in Utah to serve on juries [*McPherson vs. McKerrick*].)

Returning to Portland as a doctor, I often would meet folks who recalled with amazement that, as a little girl, I had always insisted I was going to be a doctor. Black female doctors were as common as unicorns in the "integrated" North, but professional Blacks represented the triumph over Jim Crow. They served the community despite barriers and obstacles. In those days all professionals served, but those Negro professionals understood their unique obligations as the "Talented Tenth," to "pull all that are worth the saving up." This group of professionals, while not perfect, knew they had a special obligation.

My maternal great-grandfather, J. W. Taylor, born in 1857, purchased property that is still listed on the tax rolls of St. Martin's Parish. He graduated from a land grant college during Reconstruction. As for me, with ancestors who struggled at great personal cost, why couldn't I become a doctor? My parents actively volunteered, so I became a volunteer. In high school I volunteered on "Pill Hill," the University of Oregon Medical School, and became more convinced that I wanted to be a doctor.

Stanford University was heaven on earth. It was the first time in my life I was around non-relatives like me: Black strivers with a plan. A high percentage of Stanford undergrads of all ethnicities wanted to become doctors. After biology classes, differences developed among the premeds. The fixers (surgeons) emerged. They dreamed of going in, fixing the problem, and moving on. The 1960s TV surgeons, Dr. Kildare and Ben Casey, never attracted me. I understood doctoring as relationships, not procedures—the kinds of relationships that developed over years. Among the Stanford non-surgeons, two groups developed: those who liked children and those who preferred adults.

The eighth class of the modern Brown University Medical School was a great place for me. Sandwiched between Harvard and Yale Universities, Brown set its mission to develop scientists and physicians who would serve in research, academics, and clinical practice. Many universities talk about valuing clinical care, while their leadership fears they will become "trade schools for doctors." But Brown gave support and prestige to clinical medicine and primary care, creating a niche through innovation: early clinical exposure, partnership with community hospitals, integrated curriculum, and early identification programs designed to increase opportunities for Rhode Island residents and underrepresented minority groups. The school went beyond lip service and developed an Early Identification Program with Tougaloo College, a historically Black college in rural Mississippi. Some schools embraced research and scorned clinical practice—especially primary care. At Brown, however, primary care was not the red-headed stepchild of the medical school. We partnered with community physicians from the beginning. World-class research coexisted with clinical practice.

My first clinical rotations were surgery and obstetrics. Childbirth really is a miracle, but nurses were the ones who spent most of the time in labor and delivery with the patients. For the doctor, it's nine months, then game over. Alternatively, I liked the thought of working with the same patients over years, and dealing with the challenges of diagnostic dilemmas. While in medical school, I discovered that I really did like people.

After graduation, I entered the internal medicine residency at the Los Angeles County Medical Center. Patients there taught me Spanish; adults swarmed our free clinic like law enforcement officers looking to finish off a rival after a gang shooting in the parking lot; church mothers pinched my cheeks. I was short, with freckles and an Afro; they thought I was cute. I also represented a generation with more opportunities, for me personally and for the community. The Spanish-speaking patients were euphoric with my Spanish. My Spanish wasn't that good, but it represented my attempt to connect with them as individuals. I loved seniors and became a geriatrics specialist. One of my favorite patients was a veteran of World War II's "Greatest Generation," a Nisei man who had left his internment camp to join the fight for America, who played the ukulele while waiting for me to complete prescriptions; another was the dignified Black centenarian who appreciated that I understood why being called "Honey," instead of a courtesy title, enraged her.

I liked internal medicine because it included the variety of medical conditions, the challenge of making the right diagnosis, and the promise of directing the right treatment and establishing relationships with people. Los Angeles County Hospital was one of the largest hospitals in the world, located in the immigrant gateway of East Los Angeles; it had three thousand beds in 1982–1985. After the 1994 Northridge earthquake, multiple buildings/beds were closed. A rebuilt hospital opened in 2008 with eight hundred beds; money is being raised to add two hundred additional beds.

Because it was a big county hospital, it attracted interns and residents who wanted to learn medicine by treating the sickest patients around. Attending physicians taught in morning rounds while residents in training were responsible for decision making all night long. The culture was "See one, do one, teach one." A resident from one of the more "prestigious" LA hospitals might be smart, but everyone knew that we were both smart and tough.

I first learned about the limits of my stethoscope and our frayed healthcare safety net as a resident. I happened to be on call in 1983 when the floodgates opened. The state of California had decided that Medicaid patients could no longer be treated in private hospitals. So, on the effective date of the new policy, hospitals transferred patients. Ambulance convoys arrived on our doorstep. The Red Blanket Room for critically ill patients had twelve beds and sixteen patients. More patients were to arrive. Gurneys lined the hall, then another ward, then another floor. The ambulances continued to arrive.

Triage became the most important task. We identified those patients sick enough to get a bed in the Intensive Care Unit *and* who were also likely to survive to benefit. We looked for the nursing supervisor who could be persuaded to take the extra patient once the ward was full. We expected to work hard, but we didn't expect the responsibility for making life and death decisions based on the available physical space in the unit. When one patient who needed the ICU, which was full, began to die, I became horrified. These patients had insurance, but that was not enough. The patients had caring doctors and nurses—again, not enough. We didn't have the capacity for the extra patients who lined both sides of the halls waiting for care. Despite our sincere dedication, our esteemed education, and our heroic efforts, we were unable to provide adequate, much less great, healthcare. I didn't yet understand the two healthcare systems: one with adequate doctors and nurses, the other without.

I cut my six-figure medical school debt in half by joining the National Health Service Corps upon completing my training. NHSC assigns healthcare professionals to medically underserved communities. Since I planned to practice in "the community," and could use the debt relief, this program seemed good for me. They placed me in Watts. Though Watts wasn't a safe place at night, the patients appreciated us, our work, and our commitment to serve them. My elderly Black patients still thought I was cute. Mexican patients graciously encouraged my improving Spanish. I was pregnant and waddled to the *tacqueria* where the cooks would talk about putting extra food on the *morenita*'s plate in Spanish, unaware that I understood.

The Watts Health Foundation served Medicaid and uninsured patients in clinics located in a health manpower shortage area—a healthcare desert for a million people. When called at night, I drove thirty minutes to the closest hospital, knowing that the busy ER doctor didn't have time to take care of my admitted patient. And the specialist, needing to cover multiple distant hospitals, might not be immediately available. I loved my patients and my team, and would have stayed there except for one thing: a paycheck. I'm not talking about a large salary here, but about *any* salary at all.

Six months before my assignment ended, Watts Health Foundation filed Chapter 11 bankruptcy. After receiving $2,000 in pay, we went to the end of the line of creditors. Though we weren't receiving salaries, the US Department of Health and Human Services refused to release us from our contracts. In the subsequent years, six hospitals and multiple clinics closed. Watts was, and remains, a medically underserved area because doctors don't want to work there. Even those who might want to stay there can't because of the finances. Uninsured people can't pay, and Medicaid pays too little—hostage to budget deficits. In the richest nation in the world, the problems with healthcare in Watts are beyond good intentions. Hospitals within fifteen miles offered world-class care, but might as well have been in another world.

I took a job as an employed physician at a managed care clinic in a more privileged underserved community. I worked for a "pre-paid" health plan. In addition to a paycheck, I found a system of medicine that cared for an entire group of patients rather than the individual ones I was trained to treat. The patient in the exam room was important, certainly. But the patient who didn't come to the clinic was also important. I had previously thought that medical *quality* reflected what I did with the patient I treated. But quality was redefined as how we cared for all of our patients, even if we didn't see them. I understood this to be important, too, in my relationship with my patients. How many patients got vaccinations? How many patients got mammograms? We used data to *manage* their care. When is the next available appointment for dermatology? How many physicians will we need next year given our growing number of patients? What is the best way to prevent diabetic patients from needing lower limb amputations? Were patients receiving recommended services? Where should we locate offices? Which clinics should remain open after normal business hours? Who should care for patients with AIDS? How did patients perceive their clinic experience? And so forth. "Managed care" has become an epithet, but serving a population requires data, planning, and managing. Facing the AIDS crisis in Los Angeles, we could hire an infectious disease specialist or take interested doctors out of the office to receive special training. In an area with high rates of sexually transmitted diseases, we started routine HIV testing long before it became a national recommendation.

Some argue that market-driven patient-centered policies will solve all healthcare problems. In a country that values the freedom to choose, according to the American Association of Medical Colleges, we start with forty thousand medical school applicants who like science and want to help people, and end up with a shortage of doctors, especially primary care physicians: pediatricians, internists, and family practice doctors. Medical students are free to ignore needed specialties and needy communities. The physician shortage is worse in poor neighborhoods and rural areas. Patients are not going to emergency rooms for routine care because they want to, but because few alternatives exist. The market has failed to drive new physicians to primary care. The primary care workload has increased without a corresponding increase in revenue, while specialty practice has received higher income and greater prestige for decades. So it's not surprising that more young physicians choose subspecialty practices like orthopedic surgery, dermatology, cardiology, and the like.

Why should anyone care about the shortage of primary care doctors? Not everyone will need a cardiologist or orthopedic surgeon. But everyone needs a primary care doctor—the one who determines whether back pain is muscle strain, a herniated disc, or a manifestation of widespread cancer. As we live longer, we all need the doctor who will manage health and chronic illness.

How does a system with massive resources produce a shortage of the most-needed physicians? Policymakers, medical school deans, and politicians champion primary care with words, not action. Only 37 percent of US physicians practice primary care, and the numbers are shrinking annually. In the 1990s, the Council on Graduate Medical Education predicted a shortage of primary care physicians, and in the absence of a plan, a primary care physician shortage developed. Like Topsy, the slave girl in Harriet Beecher Stowe's *Uncle Tom's Cabin*, our healthcare system "just growed," with market forces guaranteeing that affluent communities get physicians and technology. Poor communities remain under- and unserved because inner-city and rural communities can't easily recruit physicians. They cannot assume that a qualified physician will be available when the need arises.

The cost of a medical education can drive students toward high-paying specialties. When medical students consider specialties, they consider whether they can earn enough money in a medical practice that can financially support itself. Loan programs fail to bring adequate numbers into primary care, because one year's salary as a private specialist pays off the loans. It's easier to envision a self-sustaining practice as a higher-paid specialist than as a general practitioner. Significant income disparities exist between primary care and specialists—especially those who perform costly procedures like cardiology and interventional radiology—and naturally, should I ever need such a procedure, I'd hope a qualified doctor performed it. But when a subspecialist's income is two to three times greater than a primary care physician's income, it's not surprising that many medical students and residents choose specialty practice. It's expected.

And since tax dollars support medical training, one might expect a plan, a process to ensure the right mix of subspecialists and primary care physicians. Instead, we have a system where technology evolves and wins. Robotic surgery, total body scans, and FDA-approved technology are more expensive, but not more effective.

In the structured environment of a medical organization, I started working on side projects: How do we reduce diabetic amputations? We hired a specially trained diabetic nurse educator who spent extra time with high-risk patients. How do we help patients recover from hip surgery? I knew that my elderly patients got relief from hip replacement surgery, but recovery was long and slow. We tried a pilot program, offering patients extra sessions of physical therapy before surgery, starting therapy early after surgery, and using aggressive measures to prevent blood clots. We found patients walked farther earlier and had less pain. These lessons seem obvious now, but were quite innovative at the time.

The Balanced Budget Act of 1997 froze the number of Medicare-funded residency slots, incorrectly anticipating a physician surplus. Thirteen years later, the 2010 Patient Protection and Affordable Care Act will add fifteen thousand physicians by 2015. Unfortunately, the United States is still short seventeen thousand primary care physicians. This shortfall is expected to explode to forty-six thousand by 2025. As doctors get older and retire, there is not a large supply of young doctors waiting to replace them; the result will be that the severe shortage will become worse. The 2010 act increases Medicare payments for primary care physicians in underserved areas by 10 percent. What does this mean to the untrained eye? It could mean that the doctors already there will get paid 10 percent more. It doesn't necessarily mean that places with an extreme shortage will ever have a glut of primary care doctors. And studies show that communities with high ratios of specialists have higher mortality rates than communities with higher ratios of primary care physicians.

Patient-centered medical homes and accountable-care organizations may help stretch the current workforce. But the organizational and financial requirements exclude many physicians. Start-up cost estimates range from $1 million to $11 million. While the United States spends more per capita on healthcare than any other country, we lack a system to ensure an adequate workforce. The 1997 anticipated physician surplus failed to develop.

What's the solution?

My aunt, Anger Winson Gates Hudson, was a firebrand Mississippi civil rights activist. She started trying to register to vote in 1937, paid the poll tax, and kept trying to register until 1962. She wore a red dress to the Leake County courthouse for registering because she received a card saying, "The Eyes of the White Knights of the Ku Klux Klan are Upon You." She figured that if they were watching, she didn't want them to miss her. After teaching in the segregated grade school, she brought the first desegregation lawsuit in rural Mississippi. The murdered civil rights activists Michael Schwerner, James Chaney, and Andrew Goodman slept on her floor before going to Philadelphia, Mississippi. She described her life's work as "a lonely walk." Voting, education, roads, and healthcare. She spent her life "fighting the good fight."

Quality healthcare is more than an insurance card. It is more than technology. It includes caring people in all communities. Changing primary care is a lonely walk that will require the vigorous, sustained fight of many individuals. If not us, then who?

TWELVE

The Businessman

Frederick P. Beavers

I met him late Friday night after I was called by the resident to evaluate a "patient with peripheral vascular disease and foot wounds." I asked the surgical resident whether this was acute, requiring me to see the patient that evening, or whether, based on the patient's clinical condition, it could wait until the next day. The resident summarized that the patient had chronic foot ulcers, and that the formal evaluation could wait.

The next day was my vascular surgery clinic day where I saw twenty-two scheduled patients and two additional consults. I also had an off-campus commitment scheduled. So my first contact with the resident's patient from the night before was at 10 p.m. I reviewed his chart and noted that he was in his fifties and this was his third admission to a medical institution for this problem.

The first institution evaluated and treated him for gangrene. After his vascular surgical procedure and partial foot amputation, the patient was sent to a rehabilitation facility. He wasn't there very long before he had a stroke. He was transferred to our hospital for further evaluation. Shortly thereafter, the admitting service called the surgical resident to see the patient.

I met him while he lay in bed. His legs were completely wrapped in gauze and dangled from the side of the bed. He was in obvious discomfort—to the point that he could not lie all the way back and elevate his legs on the bed. He was unwilling to let me remove the gauze for a visual examination. The resident who initially evaluated the patient had seen the patient's wounds, taken photographs, and showed them to me.

I introduced myself to the new patient. Given the lateness of the hour and his distress, I didn't think he wanted to talk much.

The patient, however, kept repeating that he'd left several important responsibilities in his life unattended. He had business trips to make. He wanted to leave the hospital prior to any further testing. Given the time of night and his additional medical conditions, I thought there was a large mental disconnect on his part. But I gave him the benefit of any doubt. I told him there was no emergency to his medical problems. In fact, I would need time to obtain and review his medical records from his previous hospitalizations. He was glad to hear it. He wanted to leave the next day to put his affairs in order and make at least one business trip before any further testing or surgical procedures.

Again, I looked at the pictures of his wounds and wondered about his mental state.

As a standard practice, I do not look at patients' demographic admission sheets. But in this instance I wanted to see what type of business he was involved in that called for him to travel when he was extremely ill. The sheet stated he worked in a supervisory capacity for a board of education in one of the suburban counties that surround Washington, DC. Given this information and our conversation, I was even more confused by the educated businessman's behavior. But it was late. I sat down in a chair near the nurses' station, opened the part of the chart that contained the medical progress notes, and began writing my own surgical consultation note. My consultation notes are detailed under most circumstances. But, due to the late hour and my own lack of energy, I wrote a summary note—my review of the patient's history, my cursory exam, and the usual list of recommendations for someone who has non-healing leg wounds and poor peripheral vascular circulation.

The next day, I came to see him on my consultation rounds, and to see if his primary team of doctors had followed any of my recommendations. I found the patient sitting in bed, his feet dangling over the side. He was awake, but somnolent. I reintroduced myself and told him why I had returned. I attempted to examine him. Although I was originally called to give my opinion about his leg ulcers and foot gangrene, I noticed several concurrent abnormalities on exam. He looked malnourished, with muscle wasting, had abnormal sounds in his neck arteries, and had a heart mur-

mur. This came as no surprise, as many patients with poor circulation of the lower legs have associated heart and cerebral vascular disease. I wondered how such an educated man could have so many medical problems.

As with all of my patients, I ended the exam by looking at his legs and feet, which were still wrapped. Because his wounds were so painful, he again did not want me to remove the dressings. Unlike the night before, though, I took my time and tried to convince him that I needed to see his wounds to make a recommendation on how best to treat them. He wanted me to come back the following day. I left, hoping that the recommendations I'd written the night before would be carried out by his treating medical team.

They were not.

I came to see him daily, realizing that at some point he would relent and let me examine his feet. I also knew that the test results would return, which would allow me to decide if any therapy I could offer would help. Day after day I returned to his bedside. It took four visits for him to allow me to look at his feet. Among other things, I saw that he had advanced gangrene. The vascular lab studies revealed severe vascular occlusive disease. This combination led to my recommendation that he undergo an above-the-knee amputation. It was clear to me that he did not want to consider this option, and once again voiced his desire to go home and attend to his business.

Realizing that my persuasive powers were ineffective and knowing that, given his advanced state of poor health, he would need to come back soon, I told him that it was acceptable to leave the hospital and return when he felt comfortable with the decision for this surgical intervention. But he never left. There was difficulty finding a rehabilitation facility for a patient who could not tolerate rehabilitation. Letting him go home, unable to walk because of the gangrene, was not an option.

Once it became clear that a decision to move forward with curative procedures for his gangrene needed to be made by someone, I asked about his family support system. He told me about his sister and her daughter. Although neither was assigned power of attorney responsibility by the patient, his niece appeared to be his major source of support in making decisions. I asked that she come to visit her uncle when I would be present in order to have a substantive discussion.

I reviewed his medical conditions and pointed out the areas of gangrene and the wounds that would not heal to his niece. I incorporated his blood test results, vascular laboratory studies, and X-rays into the collaboration to help my patient—her uncle. The last part was to explain my rationale for his treatment plan: He would require an above-the-knee amputation because of his advanced gangrene and poor blood supply. In addition, his other leg was in jeopardy due to the same issue, and its future would need to be addressed soon. Once again, he stated his desire to think things over. His niece pointed out the fact that he was stubborn, and that he wanted to try standard wound care. I told them that such standard care would not work, that his wounds were beyond healing. Somehow he managed to convince his admitting physician team that he was stable enough to be discharged. He left the following day.

I received a call in my office less than two weeks later from the nursing facility requesting that he be readmitted. Given his list of medical problems, I requested that he be admitted to the medicine service, not the surgical one. The time away from the hospital had served him no good. His gangrene had progressed, and both his nutritional state and his mental status had deteriorated. Again, he refused surgical therapy. I called his sister and niece and arranged another meeting. During the meeting it became clear that the patient now bordered on mental incompetence. However, he answered enough questions appropriately that I did not pursue a psychiatric consultation. I pulled his sister and niece aside and explained to them that his condition would only deteriorate until his gangrene was dealt with definitively. His niece confided to me that, if left to his own devices, he would never consent to the amputation. I told her I would speak to him again.

The next day, I came to see him in the morning. His mood was upbeat, though I didn't know why. He said that he realized he needed the amputation and was willing to go through with it. I found time on that week's operating room schedule and placed him on it.

The day of surgery, he was in his usual poor mood, but had not changed his mind about going forward with the surgery. I performed the amputation without complications. In a few days, his emotional disposition brightened, as if the amputation of his foot had lifted his spirits. Once we observed his medical condition for four days after the amputation, I decided to try and open the artery in his opposite leg, which was successful. He was transferred to an acute rehabilitation facility the following week.

Three weeks later, he came to my office for the first outpatient office visit a new man. We discussed how difficult a patient he was, and how once he accepted the necessity of the amputation, he changed. His niece was there and agreed that he was a new man. He was participating in rehabilitation and was on his way to obtaining a prosthesis. We said our goodbyes and scheduled a return visit for the next month. On the way out, I mentioned that a friend of mine wanted me to write a chapter in a book pertaining to medicine. I did not go into details, but told him that our journey together would fit nicely into one of the sections, and that I would send him a copy when the book was published.

One evening, after being in the operating room all day, I checked my messages. His niece had called to inform me that her uncle had died. A week later, I received a pathology report. The cause of death was cardiac disease.

I tried to digest the "what precipitated the beginnings of his complicated medical course?" At some point in his life, he must have been healthy. Why didn't he take care of himself? Why did he neglect his health? After all of the procedures that took place at the outside facilities, how healthy, if at all, had he become? Or, more realistically, why did he continue to be malnourished and debilitated? These questions arise every time I am called to evaluate a person with active peripheral vascular disease and multiple medical conditions. I wondered how this man could die at such a relatively young age. I reviewed the usual factors that contribute to disparities: the patient, the doctor, socioeconomic status, educational status, insurance, healthcare facilities. I wanted to believe that better outcomes can be—and should be—achieved. Over the next few days, I analyzed his care and his outcome.

He came to me as a consult: a person with an extensive medical history who was recently hospitalized, underwent several medical procedures, and was deemed in need of physical rehabilitation before making the transition to independent living status. Given his educational background, how could he have been so ill? I'd always assumed intelligent, formally educated people would value their health.

I tried finding the answer by listening to his story. But the nonsensical statements he'd put forth were not helpful. So I turned to his closest relative. His niece simply stated that his was a case of neglect. He did not take care of himself. That answer would satisfy most, if not all, of us who attempt to cure people with long-term maladies. But settling for this answer won't help prevent the next businessman from following a similar pattern. I question why a person chooses not to take care of himself. By accepting this answer, can we feel that we have done our due diligence as doctors? In fact, we have made it easy. We can place the blame on the person and not think that it may be us, or some other variable, that led to this willful self-neglect. Maybe an interaction during his childhood or teenage years with a doctor had colored his view forever.

My career in medicine has allowed me to interact with patients from every socioeconomic level. While the prevalence of multi-organ disease is higher in lower socioeconomic groups, those with higher educational achievement and monetary incomes have significant health issues as well. The one variable I can control is my own approach. I'm a physician with the skill to diagnose and treat a complex problem. That's why I endured a general surgical residency, a trauma surgery fellowship, and a vascular surgical fellowship. I participate in clinical research and attend the important clinical meetings. I've practiced in different settings—academic, suburban group practice, public, private, inner-city. I've seen it all. But the formal training I have received did not prepare me to treat conditions tangential, but critical, to the health of individual patients. Certainly, I know the risk factors of peripheral vascular disease (smoking, high blood pressure, diabetes, high cholesterol, etc.), and how devastating these risk factors can be on the brain and heart. Attempting to address the social and behavioral factors for each patient, however, is mentally exhausting. When I realize that the patient sitting before me is there because he is unable to take care of himself, I am awed by the privilege to help, and equally frustrated when my simple recommendations for lifestyle changes are not followed.

My draw to surgery was being able to cure people with an operation. It has taken me a long time to learn that there are few cures in medicine, and even fewer in the field of surgery. I am resolved to be a manager of illness, like my colleagues in non-surgical medicine. This has forced me to reshape my self-image from hero to mortal. It has also allowed me not to become depressed when my attempts at curing someone of vascular illness fall short. I've reached the point of dealing with patients like the businessman with both humility and lowered expectations.

I've treated many patients since my encounter with the businessman—and several with similar stories. For my own sake, I've gotten to know them and their educational backgrounds. I don't do this to fill in the fields of the electronic medical record that my office has converted to, but to gain further insight into who that person is, and how he or she reached the point of such severe illness. This, I believe, will make me a better physician, and, I hope, will make them better patients.

Income and educational achievement are both underemphasized when it comes to caring for patients. We physicians would like to believe that we treat all patients equally with respect to these variables. And by doing so, we expect similar outcomes up and down income and educational lines. Then this thought yields to reality. I've learned that understanding the patient's socioeconomic and educational status leads to the individualization of patient care. Administering therapy to a high school dropout and a college-educated person in exactly the same way is doomed to fail. How a drug works may be the same for everyone (let's save this scientific and pseudoscientific debate for another place), but helping these disparately ill patients deal with the side effects, their own particular responses, and their related social conditions must be individualized. This part, naturally, gets tricky. On the one hand, treating people equally is the goal, but we can also argue that people should be treated differently, individually. That's why this paragraph is conflicted.

I'm at a loss as I look back on my interactions with the businessman. My medical training taught me to diagnose and heal at the extremes of technology and life. I followed the recommended guidelines for the treatment of his lower extremity vascular disease. The surgical procedures I performed were successful—the amputation "cured" his gangrene. And the angioplasty on his other leg allowed for its preservation, and for him to stand. But surgical success does not equal healing. The businessman, in the end, remains a statistic that bespeaks disparities in healthcare. His medical outcome was death.

THIRTEEN

Good Guys

Tim Degner

Spring 1967. I was in the fifth grade. Lyndon Johnson was the president. I was betrayed on page 278 of *This American Journey*. That was my fifth-grade American history book. I do not remember the exact sentence, but it went something like "the atomic bombs dropped on Hiroshima and Nagasaki brought the war in the Pacific to a close." I remember reading past this simple sentence. I read it again to make sure I had not misunderstood the lesson.

What bombs?

Over two decades had already passed since those bombs dropped by the time I'd read this, but little remained in the history book after page 278. The "good stuff" had been exhausted, and the remaining twenty-odd years could be telescoped into a few summary paragraphs. On page 279 the Korean peninsula was bisected on a map and a couple of sections elaborated. On the next page the strangely ursine visage of Leonid Brezhnev decorated a brief summary of our archnemesis, the godless Soviet Union. The page after that featured a rocket ship, and the one after that a blue-inked rubber stamp that listed the names of the Holly Avenue Elementary School students who had been betrayed by the book in the years before me.

The notion of atomic bombs was not new or foreign to us. Quite the opposite. We were Cold War kids. All of our dads had been in the war to some extent. The final Friday of every month, right at 10 a.m., air raid sirens sounded, and we'd all get under our desks and cover our heads and face away from the windows. Away from the blast. Every month.

There was a name for this then: mutual assured destruction, and its most telling acronym—MAD. We had nuclear weapons. Of course we did. Why wouldn't we? How else could we hold the Soviet Union at bay? In 1967 the Cold War was permanent. The Soviets were the eternal Lex Luthor to our Superman. A never-ending stalemate, each side repelled from action by the lethal potential of the other. That the Soviets would use their terrible weapons was a given. If not for our strength, we would be annihilated. For some reason they hated us, our American Way, our freedom, or so we were taught.

So I could not wait to get home to talk to Dad that 1967 afternoon. I had to hear it from him directly. It's not that he or anyone else had ever directly told me that we *hadn't* already dropped atomic weapons, and that they weren't only hypothetical risks. The very fact that these weapons were so horrible, so threatening, carried with it the implicit understanding that they had not actually been used by anyone. Good guys defend themselves; they don't act first. We were the good guys.

Just as surely as every teenager rebels against his parents, every fifth grader is a carbon copy of those same parents. I was no different—I supported the ongoing war in Vietnam; the war protestors were likely just cowards. Soon, I'd root for Nixon. So when Dad told me that the bombing of Hiroshima and Nagasaki hastened the end to the war, saved American lives, I was satisfied. But that wasn't the issue. The issue was that I wasn't told.

The issue wasn't atomic bombs. Had my text detailed the firebombing of Dresden (it didn't), I could have used that instead. Or the "relocation camps" that American ethnic Japanese were sent to, for that matter. The issue was much more basic. Who are *we*?

In 1967, the notion that I, or anyone I knew well, could be racially biased really never crossed my mind. No one in my family ever openly used a racial epithet, and my brother and I were taught that everyone was equal. My maternal grandparents were Italian immigrants, poor laborers who spoke poor English. If I were to have any context at all about racially based discrimination, my family members would likely be the victims, not the perpetrators. Even that concept was entirely hypothetical. No one ever called me a "wop" in school; until I read that term in a book, or saw it in a film, I had never even heard of it. It was a quaint anachronism, a relic of Chicago, or Boston, or New York of decades past.

The civil rights movement, to us, was a story that had ended, after having taken place elsewhere. The University of Alabama was integrated. Everyone voted. The Watts riots, a mere twenty miles away from my house, had been little more than a television special. Neither I nor anyone I knew had ever seen a "Whites Only" drinking fountain. No one I knew in Los Angeles took the bus, front or back. This wasn't our story.

Not until the Nowitzkis decided to move, that is.

The Nowitzkis lived next door. On our tract-house street, every other house was identical, with the intervening houses being mirror-image opposites. One never needed to ask where the bathroom was when visiting a friend on our street. The one distinction of the Nowitzki house was the bomb shelter in the backyard, with its large steel plate and handle covering a ladder leading to a concrete, belowground bunker. This wasn't a metaphor, but an actual bomb shelter; I could see the door from my bedroom window.

The Nowitzkis called a neighborhood meeting—the first, the only neighborhood meeting ever held in the history of Greenfield Avenue. Its purpose was to announce their intent to sell their home to a Black couple, the would-be beginning of integration of the neighborhood. My parents returned from this first, this only meeting, with a new lexicon, one I'd never before heard: "Property values will drop." "You could give *them* Beverly Hills and they'd turn it into Watts." "They have no right."

Even at age eleven I was fairly sure the "Beverly Hills/Watts" comment was not a report of a possible experiment. And I was fairly certain that race couldn't be taken into account when selling a house. True, Greenfield Avenue's inhabitants were all the same race. For the first time, I began to see why. As with Hiroshima, I asked my father if this was the case: Is it not illegal to discriminate based on race when selling your house? He replied that he thought it might be, and didn't say much more.

The Nowitzkis eventually sold their home to the Tans, a White family. There were no further neighborhood meetings, and the matter never came up again. But I think I had learned a lesson. We are the good guys, always. It isn't about what we do; it's about who we are. And when our behavior doesn't measure up . . . well, those pages don't make it into the history texts.

* * *

I'm now a practicing pediatric cardiologist and the head of a large urban pediatrics department. I also volunteer my time as clinical faculty at UCLA School of Medicine, teaching first-year students to interview actors who simulate patients. The curriculum includes a provocative 1999 study by Kevin Schulman and associates from Georgetown University in a special article in the *New England Journal of Medicine*. The authors found bias among physicians, in the form of racial stereotyping. Videotapes about a patient with chest pain were shown to the doctors in the study. The doctors were asked what they'd do next. The patients were identical: same symptoms, jobs, insurance, educational level, test results, age. Almost identical, that is; their race and gender differed. They even read the same script and spoke the same dialect of English. White male patients had extensive, technology-laden testing ordered. Black and Hispanic patients received more basic testing. Women of color received the least involved testing. White women fell in between White and Black men.

Just as I had searched that sentence about the bomb to see where I had misread, I searched the article for flaws. Something else must have been going on. Perhaps the physicians felt the racial minority patients couldn't afford the more involved tests and were trying to save them money? Maybe the White male patients were just more demanding and badgered their way to tests that should have been second- or third-line all along. No such luck. The doctors simply treated the patients differently based on their perceived race.

Glyn Lewis et al., from London's Institute of Psychiatry, published in the *British Journal of Psychiatry* in 1990, showed very similar findings among British physicians. Psychiatric patients with an identical history were given less medication and judged to be "potentially violent" more often if they were Afro-Caribbean than White. In 2000, in the journal *Social Science and Medicine*, Michelle Van Ryn showed that physicians attributed negative stereotypes to ethnic patients, such as "likely to be less educated," "less likely to be pleasant," or "likely to be less responsible." Even when factual information was available, such as a documented level of education, the stereotype still prevailed.

I know about White guilt—I'm half German. But the emotion I felt reading these studies wasn't guilt, but rather resentment. Much in the same way I imagine my father probably felt when confronted by the young me decades ago. "It's complicated!" I found myself thinking, much as my neighbors could not separate the concept of fairness from the concept of investment values on Greenfield Avenue during the late 1960s. I, like all doctors, believe that had I been a participant in that videotaped study, I would have treated all of the patients equally. I'm sure of it. (At least now that I'm aware of the study results, I would.)

It goes without saying that physicians have the best interests of patients in mind. It must be so, because, in part, we're selected for that. Alone among the professions, medicine virtually demands that aspirants to the field declare their desire to serve mankind. So, if poor outcomes suggest otherwise, the solution, in a discipline obsessed with education, is more education.

If physicians are to accept and confront prejudice, then medical—even pre-medical—educators should incorporate this into the curriculum at the earliest possible opportunity. The UCLA School of Medicine teaching in which I am involved includes the use of "standardized patients" to teach interviewing techniques. Standardized patients are actors who portray patients and who follow a script. Ask them a particular question and get a predictable answer. In other words, they are prepped to act as real patients do.

One of the patients is used to highlight the notion of cultural awareness. He is a thirty-ish Hispanic gardener with diabetes. He has health-care insurance, but no prescription drug benefits. He does not get paid time-off benefits for sick days, so he loses money if he goes to the doctor's office. He speaks broken English, but declines a translator. He has a sixth- or seventh-grade education. When he arrives at the "office," he is not taking most, if any, of his diabetic medications, and his blood sugar is very high. He lives in a multigenerational home, where his mother cooks for the family.

Interestingly, more than a few students throughout the years have stated they were offended by this portrayal. "How can a rank stereotype teach us not to stereotype?" they've asked. Other students try to teach this man about his diabetes. I hear them talk to him about his pancreas and about the "glycemic index" of the white rice he eats nightly, as his eyes glaze over. Even as I watch and take notes, preparing to counsel them on the overuse of jargon and their failure to assess the man's social dynamics, I cannot help but feel some frustration: Were he my patient, I'd likely fail with him, too. I'd get, at most, twenty minutes to spend with him, assuming he was on time, and he'd be unlikely to want to come back to the office with any degree of regularity. He'd be an "adverse outcome" and, being Hispanic, would serve as evidence for an ethnic-based dispar-ity among my own patients. I'd probably secretly hope he changed doc-tors altogether, or was replaced with a college-educated Hispanic of simi-lar age, with whom I would have a fighting chance of success.

Another actor-patient, a smoker, is White and articulate. He has no interest in quitting his habit, which frustrates the students to no end, this being their "motivational interviewing/stop smoking module." He is po-lite, even cheerful, and just loves his smokes. He has no interest in quit-ting: not for his health, the health of his daughter, not even after he's "hospitalized for pneumonia." Most of the students are annoyed by him. Many are eager to leave him to his "dirty habit." "It's his own fault," many have said out loud. What's pedagogically interesting here is that the notion of *physician bias* is illustrated by this patient, and not the one around which the *cultural competence* module is based. I often point this out to the students, but it's not in the tutor guide, and I'm not sure many of my co-instructors even see it this way. When prejudice and righteous indignation intersect, it's not a fair fight. (This may have been true for Harry Truman and Hiroshima as well, or maybe that's a stretch.)

In 2005, at the height of his popularity, comedian Dave Chappelle disap-peared. Rumors, later found to be untrue, placed him in South Africa in a mental hospital. When he resurfaced, Chappelle appeared on Oprah Winfrey's daytime talk show and addressed the rumor thusly: "Who goes to Africa for healthcare?" Indeed. Although meant in jest, Chappelle had a point. Even the harshest critics of American healthcare will admit that our healthcare, even at its worst, is not bad.

Proponents of the status quo in American healthcare often pronounce it "the envy of the world." While this is bravado—hyperbole, even—it's not entirely false. Stories of frustrated Canadians short-circuiting lengthy queues to avail themselves of American operations (for cash) abound. These stories of spectacularly successful surgeries are sometimes apocry-phal, always anecdotal, and certainly outnumber the stories of Americans going abroad for medical care by a country mile. In fact, other than homeopathic cancer treatments in Mexico, and the brief fad of "medical vacations" to India to take advantage of low physician labor costs for surgery, travel abroad for medical care is like people who win the lottery: For all the winners on record, I've never met one. It is a fact that foreign physicians clamor to train in the United States, and that the level of technology here is near the forefront, hampered only by the deliberative pace of the Food and Drug Administration.

The cost of healthcare is another matter entirely. When it comes to cost, perhaps we can use Mike Tyson's paraphrased words: No one can beat us. We Americans pay more of our GDP (gross domestic product) toward healthcare than any other nation. Whether the quality of the care we receive is worthy of its extraordinary cost is arguable. Many indexes of healthcare outcomes put us on a par with countries that spend far less. If there is such a thing as medical "value"—the quotient of outcomes divided by cost—surely that of the United States ranks below the rest of the Western world.

Mention "reform," and Americans smell a rat! Reform sounds much like its alliterative, snaggle-toothed cousin "ration," and nothing raises the collective hackles of Americans more than the notion of lining up and giving up free choice. Besides, it's a moot point: We can't afford it. Healthcare in America already uses up a greater percentage of GDP than in any other nation on earth, and in this time of newly realized fiscal honesty, we just cannot spend any more than we already are. This is as good as it gets: Famous comedians and foreign dignitaries come here for care, so it must be good, and to include the poor and disadvantaged to any greater degree would either cost too much or require those who are well taken care of to submit themselves to a bloated, faceless, bureaucratic death panel.

Of course, this is nonsense. From a purely hypothetical standpoint, we can spend whatever percentage of GDP on healthcare that we choose to. North Korea, the Chihuahua of nations, angry and pugnacious, spends perhaps 150 percent of its GDP on the military. Not that this is enviable, but no one ever questions the relative allocation of funds to healthcare compared to, say, defense. (No one other than Bill Maher, who ended up on cable television.)

Much more pertinent, though, is the notion that there is a class of Americans currently untreated that we simply cannot afford to cover at this point. We do treat them now, and in a very expensive fashion. The less integrated a patient is into a healthcare system, the more likely he or she is to receive care in that lowest of all categories of healthcare efficiency: the emergency room. In the ER, every visit is treated as though it may be the patient's one and only, which leads to a high utilization of resources. And every doctor knows this because virtually every doctor at some point trained in an institution that treated this class of patients.

Things don't end there. The well-connected also get inefficient care. My mother lives in Newport Beach, the home of *Gilligan's Island's* Lovey and Thurston Howell III, as I recall. My mother has Parkinson's disease: common, chronic, and slowly degenerative. She has a host of physicians, all with hospital privileges at a tony hospital featuring rooms with a high-rise ocean view. Last July Fourth weekend, she was admitted to the emergency department with a facial muscle spasm. While I am a pediatric cardiologist with no experience with Parkinson's, even a cursory review of some online resources told me that this was a muscle spasm, and not a stroke. The emergency room physician felt likewise and treated my mother with a single intravenous drug, Benadryl, which reversed the symptom within minutes. So far, so good. He next admitted her to the hospital due to her "weakened state." It was a Saturday, the beginning of a three-day weekend. I visited her on Sunday, and she was recovered.

She was discharged home on Tuesday, the first weekday after the three-day weekend. Over the course of three hospital days, she received only her own home medications and routine meals. She was seen once each day by a different hospitalist (a hospital-based physician who knew no more about my mother than what was written in the hospital medical record). My mother's neurologist, who manages her Parkinson's, was not on call that weekend. My parents went to visit the neurologist in her office on Wednesday. The only information she received was what my father could verbally relate to her from his eighty-seven-year-old memory, the same one that often cannot remember the name of the old movie he just finished watching.

I doubt they hospitalize, and pay for, elderly Parkinson's patients in Costa Rica or Slovenia for three days simply because it's the Fourth of July weekend when doctors aren't motivated to visit and a Medicare-esque program will pay the bill. These countries, where comedians also never go for healthcare, have outcomes similar to ours, and spend far less to achieve them.

Why does this happen? Because the reimbursement system for doctors makes no effort to dissuade it. The American healthcare reimbursement system is like kids' soccer leagues—everyone gets a trophy for showing up. If the point of medicine is almost certainly to obtain good outcomes, then it makes sense to pay for outcomes. Better outcomes, more pay. If the Spanish-speaking diabetic guy from my students' class needs more time in the office, spend it, and simply be reimbursed not for the length of his appointment, but for his eventual blood sugar outcome. This is currently not the case: "Fees" are awarded for the "services" rendered with outcomes either disregarded altogether or awarded a tiny "Pay for Performance 'tip.'"

This won't be easy. Just as my parents didn't want to see a just cause lead to a loss of equity in their home, I don't want to earn a penny less for the sake of increasing the value of US healthcare. Like every physician, I already believe I practice cost-efficient, streamlined medicine. Just like the subjects in the Schulman study knew they hadn't a shred of racial bias. ER docs won't be easily convinced that they won't be sued for ordering fewer studies. Drug companies will cry that they cannot perform the research that yields wonder drugs if they cannot reap the profits derived from "me-too" superfluous but expensive products. And doctors and patients alike will want to at least *feel* that they make their medical choices behind a closed door, unfettered by some governmental Big Brother.

Still and all, American medical care costs are too high. The causes can be agreed upon, disagreed upon, labeled ethical, political, educational, technological, legal, business, or personal in nature. Oh, and medical, too, I suppose. The solution—decreased cost—beckons from all angles, sometimes even from the ones making money (even the drug companies' employees pay high premiums). We can save tax dollars by paying less for Medicare and Medicaid; we can compete in business because employers will pay less in healthcare benefits, allowing them to better compete based on the price of their product without adding the cost of healthcare benefits; medical students and practicing physicians can learn to include cost in their medical management; healthcare systems can enjoy a return on investment in software programs and clinical programs aimed at decreasing redundancies; health insurance plans can zero in on the most expensive people and coordinate their care, especially, to decrease the overall cost. This is all before we direct any attention, at all, to the actual quality of care, no matter the cost, that anyone can expect to receive in the United States. And this is before we direct any attention to race.

And the success in reversing racial inequality in medicine recapitulates that in society at large as well: There is not much to show for all the effort. In fact, people are tired of the dialogue. It's like a family reunion game of Monopoly, a nostalgic treat at 8 p.m., but so tedious you hope someone tips over the board at 2 a.m. America is just fatigued with the moral arguments for achieving racial equality. They've stopped listening.

I firmly believe that my father's generation, in retrospect, felt they did the right thing at Nagasaki. But they obviously knew there was a moral issue—hence the deception. My neighbors in the 1960s knew what was right with respect to housing discrimination, but they weren't willing to risk their homes' values on their piety.

A wise friend of a friend liked to say, "All interest is self-interest." He went on to prove it by succumbing to his diabetes rather than give up his love of culinary excess.

As a nation, we may or may not make the decisions necessary to change the problems of access, quality, and racial disparities that we now see in medicine. We certainly won't if we fail to change the dialogue and the vocabulary that now frame the very discussion. We need to face up to what we're doing, not on page 278, but somewhere around page 10, where there's still some energy left to do something about it.

Greenfield Avenue, my childhood street in Arcadia, California, is now about 80 percent Asian. The values of the homes are five or six times what they were in the 1960s. I've been back to find that many of the homes have been remodeled and enlarged. I'd have to ask where the bathrooms are now. Although I wasn't there at the time, and cannot say for sure, I don't imagine that a second great "neighborhood meeting" happened on Greenfield. The original owners never changed their core values; they never had to. When their interests were aligned, change just happened.

FOURTEEN

There Is No Zeitgeist

Richard Garcia

The sun is out. Or else, there is no sun today. No one needs to do anything. The sun simply is, or is not, shining brightly, without respect for what we do. (During an episode of *Real Time with Bill Maher*, universal astrophysicist Neil deGrasse Tyson noted, "The sun is always out.") This assumes, of course, that we are out in the open, able to see. The zeitgeist, too, simply happens to an era. Or else it is derivative of an era, like the atmospheric winds of misfortune. Passively. And if one happens to have been born at a time when his adolescence has no zeitgeist, either he is destined for complacency or he can act as if there should be one. The latter is my case, I'm afraid. I missed the 1960s, though I was alive: a fetus when JFK was shot, an infant when Malcolm X was shot, a small child when MLK and RFK, later in that year at the height of a great zeitgeist that I missed, were shot. Rather, someone shot them, I should write. I don't remember the dénouement, April 30, 1975, the day South Vietnam fell, which was also one day after a seven-year-old boy who was to become my friend and colleague in medicine left Vietnam and his oldest sister for the next twenty-three years or so.

In my earliest memory I had hepatitis in south Stockton. My mother worked as a waitress at the defunct La Hacienda restaurant, which also maintained a tortilla factory in the back. Orange, and home alone, I remember calling her to ask if I could have a cupcake. (I was an obedient child, which wasn't to last much longer, I'll admit. Not to worry—this is not going to be a chapter about chronic liver failure, or the reality of memory. Not a chapter about the past, that is.) My pediatrician—everyone's pediatrician—took care of me as a toddler in his office across the street from what was to become my high school, and then took care of my own children across the street from my former high school. Still, some forty-six years later, he was the only doctor of *any* kind on the south side of town until he retired last year. So, if an adult living on the south side needed a doctor, she'd have to find her way to another side of town. Or else go to the neighboring town to the south.

My plan was to become a doctor and work there, the place where I developed my sensibility for everything at all. While I never considered attending college, I did, however, take all of the prerequisites with my Filipino friend. His mother said to him, "You'd better study and become a doctor, or else you'll pick asparagus like us." I never feared picking asparagus. Somehow, though, as a smart child, I thought I'd better listen to my friend's mother. Roger and I took the same courses from the seventh through the twelfth grades. When I was a senior in high school, my English lit teacher, Mr. Prato, asked to which college I was applying.

"None," I said.

With a pinched face, he asked, "What are you talking about?"

I had not considered college until that instant. Because of the place and family I came from, going to college never even popped up as a little bit of conversation. I mean, though Roger and I took all the right courses (he was obviously going to college), I didn't actually consider any subsequent academic pedigree. In any case, Mr. Prato convinced me without much effort. I prepared my application to UCLA because it was far from Stockton and its basketball team was often on TV. I asked Mr. Prato to take a look at my application essay before I sent it off.

"Why are you applying there?"

I told him.

"Why don't you apply to Berkeley?"

"Where's that?"

"It's about fifty miles from your front door."

I'd never heard of Berkeley. And in a final instant of bliss and adolescence, I asked, "Is it any good?"

I used some of Mr. Prato's Wite-Out and covered the Westwood address on the yellow envelope, changed it to Berkeley, and applied. (Even all these years later, I still wish I'd had sense enough to use a new envelope. And that I hadn't applied the Wite-Out so thick.) Nevertheless, I went to Berkeley. I decided to be a pre-med student, since this was the only path anyone had ever suggested. In the end, Roger became a computer engineer in those early atmospheric conditions of computers, while I went to medical school. He's more successful, by all accounts; however, his mother is proud of me.

While at Berkeley I took classes in Afro-American studies, Chicano studies, sociology, cultural anthropology, and other courses seemingly, at the time, outside of my pre-med efforts. I didn't formally pursue the social science interest I showed on this side of campus, on this side of my mind. Indeed, I had no obligation to take so many cultural and humanities courses as a pre-med student. No adviser looked at my years of study in these areas and asked why.

Neither did I.

In practical terms, I read Richard Wright, Ralph Ellison, James Baldwin, Alice Walker, and Toni Morrison without any sense that they might become part of *how* I was to consider medicine. Chicanos in film, Chicano history, and Chicano politics likewise remained segregated in my mind. Later, during my training in pediatrics and beyond, when I read Faulkner, Rodriguez, and Ellison again, I still could not conceive of how any of these lessons could relate to medicine, nor did any of my medical school professors or residency training faculty include this palette in any lessons I received in medicine.

Imperceptibly, I meandered through an article about race in one medical journal, then the next. I'd heard a couple of simplistic "cultural competence" lectures by that time. And then a substantive one by then US Surgeon General David Satcher. Coincident with reading a haphazard collection of insipid medical articles on race and medicine, and attending some well-meaning lectures, and the serious one by Dr. Satcher, I, too, wrote an article: "The Misuse of Race in Medical Diagnoses" for the *Chronicle of Higher Education*. This article was later reprinted in *Pediatrics*, a medical journal. Unaware of my place, I found myself now inside of a small collective of pieces about race and medicine. No zeitgeist, of course, but a small collective, like, say, a quartet at a jazz club in the Village.

I thought about a collective of chapters that might examine race and medicine insofar as serious attention could be paid to the disparities cataloged in burgeoning articles, conferences, speeches, e-mail chatter, and informal, whimsical dialogue. I gathered some friends—the authors of the chapters in this collective—and set out to enter a serious discourse, at least. Naturally, anyone listening at this point could only say one thing: "We already know about disparities. What we need are solutions. What's the answer?"

How we evaluate disparities inside the context of race in America's history seemed more apt, if less precise.

There's a bridge I haven't quite made with all this talk about disparities. I'm close, I think, and we may have created this bridge during our examination here. That is, I set out to write a book about disparities in health *care*—and not in health *status*. I understand the simple connection that poor care can result in poor status, and that poor status makes excellent care tougher to achieve. This much is easily understood, even if it isn't easily corrected. Assuming this is our goal. Whose goal, exactly, remains in question.

Like a Platonic Form, equality in healthcare, as in other places, is held before us all as something out of reach to which we can nobly aspire as we necessarily fail. But flesh exists. The wife, the husband, the daughter, the son, and the other daughter. They exist in both form and fact. Equality is the lower rung en route to humanity. Flesh—the gangrenous toe, the crushing chest, the imploding blood vessel in the brain, the pain denied—exists in the end. But not all flesh equally, however. I never like talking about these items in proportionate terms. If others' flesh is in even worse circumstances, I am not invigorated because I'm better off. No. My hunger cannot be satiated, or even influenced, by someone else's deeper hunger.

Poor health *status* is what we are all medically trained to address and, if possible, avoid. If someone smokes, we urge them to quit. We help them find cessation programs and can offer actual medical support. If someone with diabetes is obese, we encourage them to change their relationship with food for the better and to exercise, and, when medically appropriate, we can even offer surgical intervention. If a child is in pain, we can examine the ears and treat a presumed bacterial ear infection with antibiotics and offer immediate pain medication.

Poor health *care* is an indictment of our profession, and our "system." No one seriously attempts to deliver poor care. We say things like "we can improve care for everyone," thereby conflating the affluent with the poor, the White with the Hispanic, the woman with the man, the voter with the uninvited. Alas, this sounds nice.

We can talk about improving healthcare in customer service terms so that customers are satisfied the way, say, a grocery store or a large department store can keep customers, lest they spend their money at a competitor's store. But in healthcare, the *service* component of *quality* is not entirely applicable. Where there are plenty of other grocery stores— except, of course, in the "food deserts" of south Chicago or Detroit, for example—customers have the option of simply declining to spend their money there and going to a better place, even if it's more expensive.

However, this is not the case with medical care. Doctors aren't plentiful, vis-à-vis the demand, waiting for customers to choose them because of their glossy finishes or platitudes or comfortable waiting room music. Especially not when it comes to disparities in health status between the races. This is the part that has eluded me heretofore: The patient doesn't have a real choice. And if she chooses a different doctor, then the one she left is still busy, examining other people. The doctor is not out of business like Circuit City or Montgomery Ward. No. He is there. Whether he is glossy is unrelated to whether he treats the patient's lump correctly. This point is lost, it seems, in the "patient satisfaction equals patient compliance" postulation.

When race is included, the old-fashioned, dim platitudes surface, almost passively, and remind me of the zeitgeist into which I was born, even if I missed it. Cultural competence, language competence, and diversity among physicians do explain some of the variance, we can assume.

But while "cultural competence" might deliver perceived good *service*, no actual *product* quality can be claimed, let alone demonstrated. Cultural competence only addresses cultural incompetence. Language and culture are not synonyms, even if they are confused in medical and common discourse on this topic. More to the point, cultural competence isn't even possible. Doesn't even exist. If an emergency room physician or a primary care physician works in a big city, he or she simply cannot learn all of the cultural things one might need to achieve the same level of customer service—and, thereby, improved satisfaction scores, let's call them— for Russians and Mexicans, and Black people from Chicago and New York and Nigeria and Haiti, and Mexicans from Stockton and Los Angeles and San Antonio, and Chinese people from Alabama and Taiwan and San Francisco from a hundred years ago and last week.

I recently took a cultural competence course, passed it, and was able to print a page on my home printer certifying me as culturally competent, notwithstanding my childhood, education, and sensibilities. My mind. Looking a Mexican baby in the eye, touching a Thai kid on the head, calling for a translator when I don't speak Mandarin, and so forth, are the lessons available during certification.

Everyone knows that if a Frenchman comes to the ER and the physician doesn't speak French, then she needs a translator. But once access and language are controlled, as with Black people who speak English and make it to the ER, then other "cultural" things remain. This is an anemic approach to actual flesh and blood disparities, as seen in studies where Black people die in excess of their promise of life.

Diversity among physicians is rare, and is namely one of skin color and hair. Not *actual* diversity. This is the sort of thing that's highly offensive to minority people when we read it and hear it again and again. It's as if one Mexican is interchangeable with the next, or with Nigerian or Chinese or Arab physicians. This should also be highly offensive to Whites: Is an Italian so meaningfully confused with a German?

I'd call for a moratorium on disparities studies if anyone were listening. We know. They exist. Enough studies already. Now let's fix them. But how? This is an analogous suggestion I might have for public education in Los Angeles or Fresno or Chicago or Houston or Washington, DC. I could discuss fixing things with the producers of the recent documentary on health disparities who assert "social determinants"—poverty and its resulting conditions—and talk about fixing poverty, like it's been talked about ad nauseam, and ineffectively, for all time. Or else I could gather with some law school professors and talk about race and US law in this guise. I fear the same result.

I am not sick. However, this must end (later rather than sooner, one can hope). During the standard medical interaction between patients and doctors, we are taught to ask about past medical history, past surgical history, family medical history, allergies, social contexts, and to integrate this information with the physical examination—the part, more than any, that distinguishes physicians. We are also taught to include "race" in this integration. Race—so that we are sure to consider sickle cell anemia in Blacks and Tay-Sachs disease in Ashkenazi Jews. My friend innocently asked what diseases run in my family. I thought about this a couple of years ago for the first time in my life and said, "The men in my family tend to die violent deaths at an early age. I don't know what else runs in my family. These guys never get old enough for anything else to occur."

My Uncle Monchie overdosed on heroin during my sophomore year at Berkeley. At his ordinary funeral I stood there as his nephew, a child in the family, and listened to the routine sermon that included his US Army service in the Vietnam War. I stood among my cousins at the cemetery with the pile of dirt adjacent to the casket hovering over the empty space that was to be Uncle Monchie's final stop. I believe it was a priest who said a few final words. I don't remember whether a trumpeter played "Taps." I do remember two shovels poking out of the pile of dirt, waiting for the priest to finish. In the end, my eldest uncle, called Pelón, grabbed a shovel and began shoveling dirt onto the lowered casket that contained his little brother. We all stood there watching our uncle. As a curious person, I noticed things like the remaining shovel, waiting. I quickly scanned the crowd and realized that, at twenty years old, I was the next eldest male in the family present. The others were either in prison or already dead. I grabbed the second shovel and shoveled dirt with one uncle onto the other. Later that night at our house, Pelón said, "Thanks for helping me bury my brother." I did not see any uncle after that, until my Uncle Junior overdosed on heroin three Christmas Eves ago.

Of course, death by violence, or by any other hand, is, after all, death. Final. And that it "runs in my family" is troublesome to me. However, I have chosen to live in a safe city. My little children only know of these men through stories in which they are not yet interested. In my case, although I am not sick now, if all goes according to plan, I'll avoid an early violent death and live long enough to get sick. I don't expect to suffer through any healthcare disparities. I know better. What to look for. And what to look out for. My wife and children, racial minorities, all of them, will not be passive, unsuspecting prey to healthcare disparities.

I wonder what I can do to integrate the social sciences and humanities I studied in college. The lessons I learned in a violent family in a violent city. I could argue that to turn our collective attention to healthcare disparities is a smart financial move. The country pays more money in the form of taxes and insurance premiums when including disparately sick racial minorities. To disregard them would be both expensive and inhumane. But I'm not really here to argue for saving some money. Rather, I bend toward humanity. I live each day, when I can remember, in the shadow of that *Seinfeld* episode when Kramer asked Jerry to bring some Cubans back with him to New York. Jerry asked a clarifying question: "We're talking about people, right?"

FIFTEEN

Race and Medicine

Richard Garcia

My father left before I was born. Well, he didn't really *leave* because he wasn't there in the first place. What does this mean to an unconscious baby? Nothing, I thought, at first. Through the years, I reconsidered that it might mean something, but didn't know what. I thought I'd have some sort of watershed moment when my wife delivered our first baby, a daughter. I didn't. Not really, though I made room for this possibility the night she was born, thinking that, perhaps, something would come to mind. I wondered what he might think or say now that he had a grand-daughter—what he didn't think or say when I was born. My father had already died of a heroin overdose by the time our daughter was born, so he could not talk to me. Which is to say, we couldn't talk any more than we did before he died. I thought his absence would make more sense when my second child, a son, was born, I'm ashamed to say. This was not some sexist insight. But what was it?

By the time my wife delivered our third baby, a daughter, the arc was, somehow, complete: I felt nothing for my father with respect to being one myself. Time spent living without a father, coupled with being a father, became interesting to me. Other than a few humorous items, I don't talk about my childhood. I sometimes make general comments about my criminal grandfather and his brothers, my criminal uncles, my criminal cousins, and my criminal friends. I don't see these people, or this child-hood, as a vehicle, per se, to tell some *other* story. Rather, I see the childhood itself, the location of the particular language—a blend of English from school and English from my family—and the ideas, too, which stood out—and stand out—as peculiar, particular, natural ways *into* the world.

What I don't talk about is my stepfather. I don't know how on earth I can make sense of this. When I wrote those initial essays right after graduating from medical school, I wrote pieces about him. These were no good, I confess. He beat me with a belt, as early as I can remember; then he took the buckle off and created a loop where he could easily slip his hand through to hold it more securely when he beat me; I then recall a belt with metal studs, and no loop, that he wore, took off, and used to beat me; my ultimate memory of these beatings is of a brown broomstick with its bristles removed, rendering it a brown stick only, with which he beat me until the former broomstick splintered into unusable pieces that last time in the garage.

That was in the eighth grade.

Born without a father, into a criminal milieu, followed by beatings with belts, studs, and sticks. But I was smart, had a Filipino friend whose parents urged him into medicine, and was accepted to Berkeley. When I thought about *why* I should become a doctor, I couldn't help but think about what else I might do with my life once I was able to break out of adolescence. Some things interested me: books by Jean Toomer, Zora Neale Hurston, and Richard Wright that I read at Berkeley.

But what would I do?

I thought I might go to graduate school and get a PhD in some area of study. My sociology professor, who knew I was considering medical school, said, "We have enough sociologists. What we need are doctors out there helping people."

What I wanted to *do*, it seemed, was become a teacher, a pediatrician, or a child psychologist. These seemed interchangeable to me then.

As a pediatrician, in a way, I could live the narrative structure of my life that begins with an impossible life and inadvertent classes, and concludes with board certification in pediatrics. While I hesitate to publicly admit this (I suppose this next part doesn't sound as bad as the other things I've written here), I didn't enjoy clinical medicine as much as I'd hoped. Whether working in a pediatrics office, an urgent care center, or an ER, I remained interested in those college courses rooted in race, inequality, the dissonant expression of my own role in how I could make sense of the brutality, the medicine, the social science. I learned about health disparities when comparing different races of Americans, wrote some articles of my own, gave some speeches, and examined how I could couple my interest in race and medicine so that it might be congruent with my life's personal narrative structure.

My closest friend in adulthood, a rhetorician whom I met at Berkeley, is the one who first clarified this for me. He noted that Malcolm X, as a child, wanted to become a lawyer so that he could help his people.

"Malcolm X didn't attend law school, but, in the end, lived a life using his talent to help his people. Malcolm realized his 'narrative structure,'" my friend said to me. "While he didn't become a lawyer, he did what he set out to do, in fact. That's what you're doing. You've realized your dream. Not many people get to realize their childhood dream."

My friend, the rhetorician, died a couple of years ago. Some other friends and I attended the National Communications Association annual convention and presented a panel discussion in his memory. Since we couldn't just eulogize our friend, we gave speeches on aspects of his area of study: the rhetoric of the Black church. For my part, I spoke about the role of the audience. I talked about the pews, as it were. I also told them about my friend's great loves: Häagen-Dazs, words, and Black people. I told the audience of professors that my friend and I had a twenty-two-year conversation that didn't end until his death. One or the other of us would need to hang up the phone to teach a class, work an ER shift, or work on a chapter. I live without my friend now. No one to help me and my wife make sense of our questions about our children's education, our isolated suburban location, my identity as a Mexican who's never been to Mexico, my role as a doctor.

I'm alone here, in a way.

Another friend, Richard Rodriguez, recently offered this when I mentioned my own disappointment with life: "This is the source of your greatness and also your entrance into the full flush of middle age—the discontent. Without discontentment, you would never write or listen to music in your mind or dream. She is your best muse—Disappointment—but you never know how to properly greet her."

Where I am in life is extraordinary for middle-aged men in my family, who routinely die young, hard deaths. Beyond this point in life has always been out of the question.

My friend, the rhetorician, lived a miserable final year or two. His health quickly worsened from complications of his first love: food. He knew I was working on a book about health disparities, and would share his own stories in medicine with me. At first I listened and tried to help by talking with his doctors, going with him to appointments, explaining his options to him, and answering his questions. I did what I could. Without noticing, I became more emotionally involved than I would have thought as a trained physician. After all, he was my friend. In the final weeks, I asked one of my medical school classmates, a nephrologist, how he thought I should help coordinate my sick friend's terminal care. My classmate said, "Be his friend. Ask him, 'How you doin' today?'"

He died. I struggle without my dead friend's consultation. He is not the reason I'm writing these chapters. Nor are my dead-too-early grandfather, father, and uncles. This collection of sentences, I suppose, is a version of the dissonance of my life as a doctor.

My struggle with race and medicine is, perchance, my *raison d'être*.

Three babies: girl, boy, girl. Father, husband, son, brother, nephew, cousin, uncle, doctor. I'm a man in my family, still alive, in the end.

Not alone, then, as I look around: my wife, our three children, my childhood friends, my adult friends, and my family—the ones who remain.

I don't suppose I do much beyond exist among the others. However, as it turns out, this is my greatest accomplishment, I'm sad to admit.

My eldest daughter, a ninth grader, and I discuss Chinese history or Greek mythology. I play tennis with my son, a sixth grader, who is already better than me in so many ways, in my expert opinion. The six-year-old: I listen to her narratives, which are already more fantastic than my own. My wife and I worry about their health, their happiness.

With respect to race and medicine, in an earlier chapter here, I asked myself Montaigne's question: *What do I know?* I suppose I also ask my own question: *What can I do?*

Bibliography

Alexander, Michelle. *The New Jim Crow: Mass Incarceration in the Age of Colorblindness.* New York: The New Press, 2010.

Benjamin, Ruha. "A Lab of Their Own: Genomic Sovereignty as Postcolonial Science Policy." *Policy and Society* 28 (2009): 341–55.

Bullard, Robert D. *Dumping in Dixie: Race, Class and Environmental Quality.* Boulder, CO: Westview Press, 1990.

Burchard, González E., et al. "The Importance of Race and Ethnic Background in Biomedical Research and Clinical Practice." *New England Journal of Medicine* 348 (2003): 1170–75.

California Newsreel, available at http://www.unnaturalcauses.org.

Cheng, Gang. "Clinical Review of Iressa for the Treatment of NSCLC." *Chinese Journal of Clinical Oncology* 2, no. 5 (2005): 829–33.

Cho, A., J. Martin, et al. "Incorporating Discussion of Cultural Diversity throughout the First-Year Medical Curriculum." *Journal of the Association of American Medical Colleges* 74, no. 5 (1999): 582–83.

DeMouy, Jane. "The Pima Indians and Genetic Research." http://diabetes.niddk.nih.gov/dm/pubs/pima/genetic/genetic.htm (accessed June 27, 2012).

Duster, Troy. "Ancestry Testing and DNA: Uses, Limits—and Caveat Emptor." In *Race and the Genetic Revolution: Science, Myth and Culture,* edited by S. Krimsky and K. Sloan. New York: Columbia University Press, 2010.

———. "Comparative Perspectives and Competing Explanations: Taking on the Newly Configured Reductionist Challenge to Sociology." *American Sociological Review* 71 (February 2006): 1–15.

———. "Human Genetics and Human Taxonomies: Fluidity, Continuity and Transformations." *Transforming Racial Images: Analyses of Representations,* proceedings of the Twelfth Kyoto University International Symposium, Kyoto, Japan (2009): 81–102.

———. "The Molecular Reinscription of Race." *Patterns of Prejudice* 40, no. 4–5 (November 2006).

———. "Race and Reification in Science." *Science* 307 (February 18, 2005): 1050–51.

Friedrich, Mary Jane. "Using EGFR Status to Personalize Treatment: Lung Cancer Researchers Reach a Milestone." *Journal of the National Cancer Institute* 101, no. 15 (2009): 1039–41.

Fujimura, Joan H., and Ramya Rajagopalan. "Different Differences: The Use of 'Genetic Ancestry' versus Race in Biomedical Human Genetic Research." *Social Studies of Science* 41, no. 1 (2011): 5–30.

Fullwiley, Duana. "The Biologistical Construction of Race: 'Admixture' Technology and the New Genetic Medicine." *Social Studies of Science* 38, no. 5 (2008): 695–735.

———. "The Molecularization of Race: Institutionalizing Human Difference in Pharmacogenetics Practice." *Science as Culture* 16, no. 1 (2007): 1–30.

Gibson, Greg, and G. P. Copenhaver. "Consent and Internet-Enabled Human Genomics." *PLOS Genetics* 6 (June 24, 2010). http://www.plosgenetics.org/article/info:doi/10.1371/journal.pgen.1000965 (accessed August 8, 2012).

HUGO Pan-Asian SNP Consortium. "Mapping Human Genetic Diversity in Asia." *Science* 11 (December 2009): 1541–45.

Jang, Jae-Sik, et al. "Meta-Analysis of Cytochrome P450 2C19 Polymorphism and Risk of Adverse Clinical Outcomes among Coronary Artery Disease Patients of Different Ethnic Groups Treated with *Clopidogrel*." *American Journal of Cardiology* 110, no. 4 (August 15, 2012): 502–8. http://dx.doi.org/10.1016/j.amjcard.2012.04.020 (accessed August 9, 2012).

King, H., and M. Rewers. "Global Estimates for Prevalence of Diabetes Mellitus and Impaired Glucose Tolerance." *Diabetes Care* 16 (1993): 157–77.

Kolata, Gina. "New Treatments and Questions." *International Herald Tribune*, April 21, 2010.

Komaromy, M., K. Grumbach, et al. "The Role of Black and Hispanic Physicians in Providing Health Care for Underserved Populations." *New England Journal of Medicine* 334, no. 20 (1996): 1305–10.

Marks, Jonathan. "Science, Samples and People." *Anthropology Today* 26, no. 3 (June 2010): 3–4.

Mok, Tony S., et al. "Gefitinib or Carboplatin-Paclitaxel in Pulmonary Adenocarcinoma." *New England Journal of Medicine* 361, no. 10 (2009): 947–57.

Pickle, L. W., et al. "The New United States Cancer Atlas." *Recent Results in Cancer Research* 114 (1989): 196–207.

Pierce, Jennifer L. *Gender Trials: Emotional Lives in Contemporary Law Firms.* Berkeley and Los Angeles: University of California Press, 1995.

Proctor, Robert N. *Cancer Wars: How Politics Shapes What We Know and Don't Know about Cancer.* New York: Basic Books, 1995.

Reinhard, Karl J., et al. "Understanding the Pathoecological Relationship between Ancient Diet and Modern Diabetes through Coprolite Analysis." *Current Anthropology* 53, no. 4 (2012): 506.

Risch, Neil, et al. "Categorizations of Humans in Biological Research: Genes, Race and Disease." *Genome Biology* 3, no. 7 (July 1, 2002): 2007.1–2007.12.

Séguin, B., et al. "Genomic Medicine and Developing Countries: Creating a Room of Their Own." *Nature Reviews Genetics* 9 (2008): 487–93.

Séguin, B., et al. "Genomics, Public Health and Developing Countries: The Case of the Mexican National Institute of Genomic Medicine (INMEGEN)." *Nature Reviews Genetics* (2008): S5–S9.

Sharf, Barbara F., and Richard L. Street Jr. "The Patient as Central Construct: Shifting the Emphasis." *Health Communication* 9, no. 1 (1997): 1–11.

Siegel, Karen, et al. "Finding a Policy Solution to India's Diabetes Epidemic." *Health Affairs* 27, no. 4 (July 2008): 1077–90.

Steingraber, Sandra. *Living Downstream.* New York: Random House, 1997.

The Sullivan Commission. *Missing Persons: Minorities in the Health Professions. A Report of the Sullivan Commission on Diversity in the Healthcare Workforce.* 2004. http://www.aacn.nche.edu/media-relations/SullivanReport.pdf.

Sze, Julie. "Gender, Asthma Politics, and Urban Environmental Justice Activism." In *New Perspectives on Environmental Justice: Gender, Sexuality, and Activism*, edited by Rachel Stein. New Brunswick, NJ: Rutgers University Press, 2004.

————. *Noxious New York: The Racial Politics of Urban Health and Environmental Justice.* Cambridge, MA: MIT Press, 2006.

Tangwisutijit, Nantiya. "Genetic Research Raises Thorny Ethical Issues." *The Nation* (Thailand), May 1, 2005.

Von Hoffman, Nicholas. "The Rich Get Thinner, The Poor Get Diabetes." *New York Observer.* http://observer.com/2006/01/the-rich-get-thinner-the-poor-get-diabetes-2/ (accessed July 26, 2012).

Wang, Jian, et al. "The Diploid Sequence of an Asian Individual." *Nature* 56 (November 6, 2008): 60–65.

Zamisak, Nicholas, and Jeanne Whalen. "Cancer Drug Helps Asians Even as It Fails in Other Groups." *Wall Street Journal*, May 4, 2005.

Zweifler, J., and A. M. Gonzalez. "Teaching Residents to Care for Culturally Diverse Populations." *Academy of Medicine* 73, no. 10 (1998): 1056–61.

Contributing Authors

Frederick P. Beavers, MD
Chief of Surgery
Southern Maryland Hospital

Sylvia Gates Carlisle, MD, MBA
Managing Medical Director
Anthem Blue Cross California

Tim Degner, MD, FACC, FAAP
Chief, Department of Pediatrics and Pediatric Cardiology
Kaiser Permanente Los Angeles Medical Center
also: Assistant Clinical Professor of Pediatrics
David Geffen School of Medicine
University of California at Los Angeles

Troy Duster, PhD
Chancellor's Professor, Sociology Department
University of California at Berkeley

Donna Elliott, MD, EdD
Associate Dean for Student Affairs
Keck School of Medicine
University of Southern California

Richard Garcia, MD
Pediatrician
California
Contact at jazzprose@gmail.com

Jorge A. Girotti, PhD
Associate Dean and Director
Admissions and Special Curricular Programs Director
Hispanic Center of Excellence in Medicine
also: Assistant Professor, Medical Education
University of Illinois College of Medicine

A. Pérez, PhD
Associate Professor, Department of English
University of Nevada Las Vegas

Jennifer L. Pierce, PhD
Professor, Department of American Studies
University of Minnesota

Enrique D. Rigsby, PhD
President/CEO
Rick Rigsby Communications
also: Former faculty member, Department of Communication
Texas A&M University

Brian D. Smedley, PhD
Vice President and Director
Health Policy Institute, Joint Center for Political and Economic Studies
Washington, DC

Myrtis Sullivan, MD, MPH
Adjunct Associate Professor, Community Health Sciences (retired)
School of Public Health
University of Illinois at Chicago